the purpose pursuit

the purpose pursuit

8 steps to the life you've been searching for

HANNAH MILLER

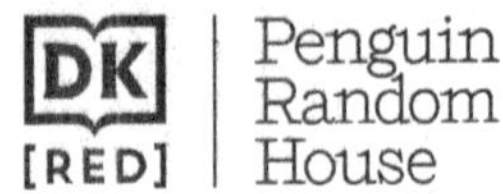

First published in Great Britain in 2025 by
DK RED, an imprint of
Dorling Kindersley Limited
20 Vauxhall Bridge Road, London SW1V 2SA

The authorised representative in the EEA is
Dorling Kindersley Verlag GmbH. Arnulfstr. 124,
80636 Munich, Germany

10 9 8 7 6 5 4 3 2 1
001–350894–Dec/2025

Cover design by Sarah Christie

Shutterstock.com: 22 TREE HOUSE 6-7, 8,16,38,64,92,110,142,188,214
(Infographic Reference)
Cover images: Front and Back: **Shutterstock.com:** 22 TREE HOUSE (Infographic Reference); Back Flap: **Mustard Yellow Photography**

A CIP catalogue record for this book
is available from the British Library.
HB ISBN: 978-0-2417-5633-1
Printed and bound in the United Kingdom

www.dk.com

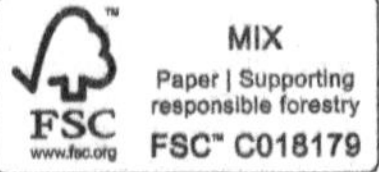

This book was made with Forest Stewardship Council™ certified paper – one small step in DK's commitment to a sustainable future.
Learn more at www.dk.com/uk/information/sustainability

Praise for The Purpose Pursuit

'A compassionate companion for anyone seeking to discover their true purpose'
Zoe Clark-Coates MBE, entrepreneur, and author

'This book puts an arm around you and shows you what's possible for your work and life'
Graham Allcott, author of *How to be a Productivity Ninja*

'Smart, grounded, and super practical. A proper reset if you're feeling off track'
TJ Power, neuroscientist and author of *The Dose Effect*

'This is a book that invites transformation through grounded, actionable steps'
Chris Guillebeau, author of *Time Anxiety*

'Packed with relatable examples and applications to weave purpose into the fabric of your everyday life'
Jo Hargreaves, psychotherapist

'Some books you read, and some books read you. This book is a beautiful tool for personal development and change'
Professor Nick Harding OBE, Chief Medical Officer

'Many books promise to change your life, but The Purpose Pursuit may well just do that'
Rachel Hughes, pastor and co-founder of The Orchard Women

Contents

Introduction

There's something deeply human about the search for purpose. It's a question as old as time itself: "What am I here for?" For some, this question burns brightly from a young age, shaping choices and direction. For others, it lingers in the background, waiting for the right moment to ask for attention. For others still, it's life's hardest moments – grief, disappointment, upheaval – that thrust the question to the forefront, demanding answers we might not feel ready to give.

Yet, for many of us, the idea of purpose feels elusive – like a slippery eel that we can't quite grasp. Or worse, it feels elitist, as though it's reserved for the lucky few who seem to have it all worked out. And so, to avoid disappointment, we lower our expectations. We reduce purpose to productivity, throw ourselves into work, make one small compromise after another, and settle for a life that is more ordinary than extraordinary. I've seen clients who, despite the appearance of outward success, feel an unshakable sense of emptiness, trapped in careers that drain them, commitments that weigh them down, and routines that leave them uninspired. They tell me they should be happy, yet something vital is missing. I've also seen clients who feel as though life has asked too much of them, whether through circumstance, obligation, or sheer exhaustion. Over time, they shrink back, believing they have little left to offer. They settle for familiarity rather than fulfilment, convincing themselves that this is simply how life is meant to be. But beneath it all, there's a quiet resentment, a fatigue that runs deep, and a sense that somewhere along the way they lost themselves.

I've worked in training and development for over 25 years, and for the past decade I've been a full-time coach, guiding hundreds of people through my Purpose Pursuit coaching course. Time and again, I've witnessed the transformation that takes place when someone steps into a life of purpose. They wake up with a renewed sense of direction, energized by a future they are actively shaping. Yes, life still comes with its challenges and responsibilities, but something shifts within them. They rediscover their confidence, their relationships deepen, and their actions – whether in their career or personal life – feel meaningful again. I've seen people finally make bold decisions they had been avoiding for years, step into roles that align with their values, and find the courage to redefine what success looks like on their own terms. Instead of merely existing, they begin to fully engage with life, choosing growth over stagnation, intention over autopilot, and possibility over resignation.

And so, what if purpose wasn't just for the select few? What if it wasn't about a single, grand calling or a once-in-a-lifetime revelation? What if, instead, purpose was something we could *build*, something that evolves, shifts, and takes shape over time? And what if your unique purpose wasn't some external prize to be won, but the sum of your talents, personality, experiences, and values – something already within you, waiting to be uncovered? This book, the culmination of countless hours of coaching and years of lived experience, is here to help you do just that: uncover and build a sense of purpose that is not a distant, elusive ideal but something practical, evolving, and deeply personal. This book will guide you towards clues that help you better understand yourself: the unique strengths and passions that drive you, the values you hold dear, and the life you want to lead. Purpose is not just about discovering what you're here to *do*, but who you're here to *be*.

Purpose is...

When I was a little girl, one of my absolute favourite books was *The Owl Who Was Afraid of the Dark*.[1] Plop, a young barn owl (who by nature is meant to be nocturnal), is afraid of the dark. Because of his fear, he refuses to go out in it or hunt with his parents. But throughout the story, Plop meets different people who each reveal a new side of the dark, one he had never considered before. They help him see that dark is kind, dark is necessary, and dark is fun. Now, I'm not saying people are *afraid* of purpose, but I do think it can feel so consuming and abstract that we sometimes avoid it. We assume it's too big, too complex, or meant for someone else – someone more certain, more confident, and more clear about their path. But just as the owl in the story learnt to see the dark in a new way, I want to offer you a fuller, more attainable definition of purpose – one that makes it feel less like an impossible quest and more like something real, something that's *yours*. Because purpose is powerful, purpose is holistic, purpose is for all of us – and purpose is a pursuit.

Purpose is Powerful

A sense of purpose has been proven time and again to make life better. Studies have shown that having a clear sense of purpose is linked to improved mental and physical health, greater resilience, and even longer life expectancy.[2] Knowing who we are at our best and getting to live that out daily also acts as an essential safeguard against burnout, crucial in a time when burnout is at an all-time high.[3] When we have a sense of purpose, it boosts our wellbeing and we're more likely to feel fulfilled, engaged, and motivated towards our goals.[4] Neuroscientific research supports this, indicating that living with purpose activates the brain's reward system, leading to increased wellbeing and lower stress levels.[5]

But beyond this compelling data, I know from my own life that when we are living in alignment with our purpose, we feel the difference in our daily lives. I've seen in my own journey how stepping into work that truly resonates with who I am has brought clarity, energy, and a deeper sense of fulfilment. I've also witnessed it in my clients, watching them move from feeling stuck and unmotivated to living with greater confidence and conviction. We all know what it's like to go through the motions, feeling disconnected from what we're doing. And we also know how different it feels to be deeply engaged, to wake up with a sense of direction, to be doing something that connects with who we are and who we were made to be. Purpose is powerful: it transforms our lives from ordinary to extraordinary.

Purpose is Holistic

One of the biggest myths about purpose is that it's synonymous with career. Sadly, I've seen far too many books reduce purpose to our paid work. While work can be a powerful vehicle for purpose, it is not the whole picture.

If we define purpose solely through work, we create a fragile foundation – one that ties our identity to what we do rather than who we are. But what happens when jobs change, careers shift, or retirement comes? If purpose is only about work, then it becomes something temporary, something that can be lost. I've worked with clients who have spent years climbing the career ladder, only to reach the top and feel an unsettling emptiness because their sense of purpose was tied entirely to their job title. I've also coached people who, after stepping away from long-held roles due to redundancy, retirement, or life changes, found themselves questioning their worth.

True purpose is bigger than a job title. It weaves through every aspect of life: our relationships, passions, beliefs, contributions, and the unique way we move through the world. It's not confined to office walls or pay cheques. It's something deeper, something enduring. This book will help you uncover what truly matters to you, beyond a job title or society's expectations.

Purpose is For All of Us

Perhaps the biggest barrier to living with purpose is the belief that it's only available to a few of us. That it belongs to people who have extraordinary talent, wealth, or a specific calling. That it's reserved for those who change the world in dramatic ways. But purpose isn't just for the people who start global movements or write bestselling books. It's for the parent raising a child with love and care. It's for the teacher who invests in their students. It's for the person who brings kindness into their workplace, who serves their community, and who shows up for their friends.

I know this because I once believed purpose had to be something huge, something that would completely redefine my life. I searched for it for years, thinking it had to be a singular, extraordinary calling. But the moment I stopped chasing an elusive idea of purpose and instead focused on aligning my daily life with what truly mattered to me, everything shifted. I discovered that purpose isn't about waiting for a lightning bolt moment, it's about making intentional choices, one by one. That discovery didn't just shape my own life, it also became the foundation of my coaching work.

Purpose is for *you*. It's not about grand gestures – it's about aligning your life with what truly matters to you. And it's not something you have to wait for; it's something you can build, step by step, starting exactly where you are.

Purpose is a Pursuit

Though in many ways this book will take you on a journey, I prefer the connotations of the word "pursuit" – it has more energy and intention, plus the alliteration is a nice bonus. But let me be clear: developing purpose in our lives does involve movement, direction, and, well... a journey. Most of us won't hear an audible voice, receive a letter from Hogwarts, or wake up one day with a crystal-clear mission etched across the sky. And there's the myth that there's only one "right" path, and that if you don't find it you've failed.

Purpose isn't about making one perfect decision, it's about making intentional choices, learning as you go, and refining your direction over time. Purpose unfolds, revealing itself in layers through experiences, questions, and choices. Sometimes, it's a slow realization; other times, it's sparked by a moment of clarity. But it's always something we move towards with effort and intention, not something that simply lands in our laps. So, while I might use the word "journey", know this: purpose isn't a destination, it's a pursuit. And you're already on the way.

How to Use This Book

The Purpose Pursuit is designed to act as your roadmap – one that you actively engage with. It's organized into chapters representing different stages of exploration and growth. Through a mix of reflection, research, exercises, and real-life examples, you'll be guided through key aspects of discovering and living out your purpose:

- **Taking stock:** reflecting on life right now, what's good, and what needs to change
- **Understanding yourself:** exploring your strengths, values, and defining moments
- **Identifying roadblocks:** understanding how we self-sabotage, through burnout, impostor syndrome, comparison, mindset shifts, and people pleasing
- **Taking action:** bringing clarity to what matters most and turning ideas into tangible next steps

Each chapter strikes a balance between reflection and action, ensuring you don't get stuck in overthinking without direction or leap into action without focus. I've drawn from the best parts of my work and personal experience to give you the strongest foundation for finding your purpose. Each chapter contains the following elements:

Concepts and Learning

I didn't want this book to be just another fluffy "You're unique and have a special purpose" pep talk, something that feels good in the moment but lacks real substance. Inspiration is important, but without a foundation of truth, it fades fast. That's why I've worked hard to ground every concept in this book in solid research. I've pored over books, journals, and studies to ensure that what you're reading isn't just feel-good rhetoric, but a roadmap built on real understanding and insight. Yes, you *are* unique. Yes, you *do* have a purpose. But to truly uncover and live it, you need more than just motivation: you need facts, science, and research to guide you forward. And that's exactly what you'll find here.

Stories and Insights

Having said all that, a book filled with research and data alone isn't enough. Facts inform, but stories transform. When I lead workshops or give talks, what truly resonates with people – the moments that stick – aren't just the studies or statistics, but the stories and anecdotes that bring them to life. That's why this book isn't just packed with knowledge, it's also deeply personal. Purpose isn't a theoretical concept: it's a human experience. And human experiences need the human element. In each chapter, you'll find glimpses of my own journey (because, let's be honest, I'm still figuring this out too) alongside real case studies from my coaching. Drawn from actual client sessions (with names changed), these examples aren't just shared for inspiration; they're here to help you see yourself in them, and to remind you that you're not alone in this. When you read these stories, you'll feel a connection. You'll feel understood. And from that place, you'll be able to make real, meaningful progress towards your own purpose.

Reflections and Activities

Understanding is important, and feeling understood is important. But neither means much if we don't *do* something about it. That's why each chapter nudges you towards action – but not before you've taken the time to reflect.

By nature, I'm a get-on-with-it kind of person. I like momentum. But I've learnt (sometimes the hard way) that real, meaningful progress doesn't happen without pausing first. Everything about the way the world works pushes us to move at a hundred miles an hour, but this stuff matters, and giving it time and space is worth it.

Reflection isn't passive. It's where you dig beneath the surface, questioning assumptions, examining core beliefs, and making sense of what you know. It's about connecting the dots between ideas that might seem unrelated at first but together reveal something deeper. It's the hidden work that makes the visible work easier.

So, you're going to want a journal. Throughout this process, I'll ask you questions that make you stop and think, followed by structured activities designed to help you plan and act. And because I know some of us love a clear framework (me included), this book is packed with practical tools to help organize your thoughts into something real – something you can actually do. Because let's be honest, that's why you're here.

Key Takeaways

Each chapter ends with a short summary, because life is busy and none of us have perfect memories. These takeaways give you the essentials: the big ideas from the chapter, the nuggets you can actually use in your life (or pass on to a friend), and the facts to help you navigate your own path or spark meaningful conversations. And most importantly, they hold the thoughts I hope will come back to you in moments of disappointment, disillusionment, or when you simply need a little reminder of what truly matters.

Time to Begin

This is not a book to passively read and then forget. It's a book to engage with, reflect on, and return to as you grow and evolve. Take your time. Use a journal. Be honest with yourself.

I didn't write this book as someone who has always had purpose figured out. I've wrestled with the same questions, experienced seasons of uncertainty and pain, and navigated my own shifts and pivots. What I've learnt – both through my own story and through coaching others – is that purpose is not a fixed destination. It's a pursuit. A dynamic, evolving process that requires courage, reflection, and action.

So, as you start to read this book, my encouragement to you is this: park your fears. Dare to hope. Stay open. Stay curious. And most importantly – commit to action. Because purpose isn't something you wait for, it's something you build, one step at a time.

Let's get started.

Chapter One

The Route

Discover Where You Are Now

The journey to discovering your purpose begins right where you are.

One Sunday morning, while my sons were at rugby training, I decided to go for a jog – or more accurately, a walk with some jogging – through the nearby fields. It was a beautiful hot day, and at a certain point I turned back, thinking I'd retrace my steps. Simple, right? Except I somehow ended up miles off course. With no landmarks in sight and Google Maps confirming my hopelessly lost state, I was rescued by Jill, a kind stranger who not only helped me get my bearings but also walked me all the way back. Turns out that my terrible sense of direction was only part of the problem; how can you find your way to where you want to be when you don't even know where you are? The same can be said of life.

You might be reading this book because you want your life to be on course, headed in the right direction, full of purpose, energy, and fulfilment. You may need clarity on your future direction, and want to know where to head next. And if you're anything like me, you just want the answers. Give me the steps, give me the plan so I can just charge ahead and get on with it. But we must first take stock of where we are and find our bearings so that we can be sure we are on the right track. Let me take you back to my Sunday morning run for a moment; I didn't know where I was and ploughed on regardless, and even though I was just a little bit off track to begin with, I ended up nowhere near where I thought I would be. Being even one degree off course can have quite an impact on your final destination – I am testament to that! Experts in air navigation have a rule of thumb known as the 1 in 60 rule. It states that for every degree a plane veers off course, it misses its target destination by one mile for every 60 miles it flies. This means that the further you travel, the further you are from where you intended to be. So, if you deviate off course by just one degree when flying around the equator, you'll land almost 500 miles off target!

Similarly, life doesn't go off track in a single, dramatic moment – it happens gradually, often without us realizing it: a small compromise here, a distraction there, a season of busyness that pulls us away from what really matters. Sometimes it's external forces such as unexpected life events, but other times it's internal, a quiet drifting caused by neglecting what fuels us, losing sight of our values, or ignoring the nagging feeling that something isn't quite right. And the thing is, you don't always notice when you're just a little off track. Everything still looks okay. Life is full, responsibilities are met, and you keep going. But over time, that small degree of misalignment adds up, and suddenly you find yourself 500 miles off target. One day, you wake up and wonder: how did I get here? Why does this not feel like the life I was meant to live?

This is why reflection matters. Before we can move forward with clarity, we need to pause. We need time to assess where we are right now, acknowledge what's working and what isn't, and make conscious choices about where we go next. It's not about dwelling on past mistakes or regrets; it's about course-correcting before we end up too far from where we truly want to be. Before we can continue on a clear path and move towards a life full of purpose, we need to take the time to orientate ourselves and identify what life looks like right now, decide what's working and what isn't, and chart a course from there.

Understanding the Seasons: The Bigger Picture

I adore the sunshine, and if it was left up to me I think I might opt for a perpetual summer. But in reality, I know that's not a good thing. A never-ending summer would lack the necessary changes to promote growth cycles, rest periods, and the natural rejuvenation that comes with different seasons. It would end up causing exhaustion, stagnation, and unfulfilled potential.

The same can be said about how we view our lives. I think it's appealing to most of us to have a life that could be metaphorically called a continuous summer – full of the best bits, the times of fruitfulness, fun, and freedom. Give me holidays, happiness, promotions, birthdays, new beginnings, and celebrations and I'll take a hard pass on the daily grind, tears, redundancies, deaths, endings, and disappointments, thank you very much. However, deep down, we know that isn't what life is or indeed should be. Without the other seasons, we miss the essential moments of reflection, rest, and renewal that are necessary for growth and real fulfilment. The best lives involve *all* this stuff. Purposeful lives feature all four seasons. Let's consider some definitions of the seasons of life, to help you identify which one you're in right now.

Spring: The Season of New Beginnings

I know I said I love summer, but spring is equally wonderful, too. In our lives, it signifies the season of growth, renewal, and fresh opportunities. It could be the early stages of a career or role, a budding relationship, a time of personal development, a new baby, or the launching of a new project. To use the analogy of a new home, perhaps spring is mid-renovation, when the foundations are in and you're building a new footprint. It's the season when we see signs of life, with fresh shoots appearing that show us that the seeds we planted and the work we did behind the scenes are starting to show their worth.

If you're in this season, you're ready to take hold of something new, and the change you hoped for is pretty much on the horizon. It's quite a stretching time because the new things you are doing are still finding their feet, but it's optimistic and filled with possibility. The daylight is increasing, providing an energy that invites us to embrace change, step out of our comfort zones, and take risks. It's a time when the foundations we've laid begin to show real potential, even if the full picture isn't clear yet. This season rewards our trust in the process, as we start to see the fruits of our efforts. It carries the promise of what's to come, and a gentle reminder that every season of life brings its own unique beauty and potential.

Summer: The Season of Growth and Expansion

Summer means progress, productivity, and energy. It's the time for building momentum, leaning into a season where you'll see returns on your previous investment. To continue the new home analogy, this might be the season where you're plastering the walls, decorating, and seeing the renovation take shape. Other real-life summer season examples include being content and effective in your work role, being in an established phase of a relationship, the so-called "golden years" of parenting, or being at the peak potential stage of a project.

You're not just budding anymore, you're flourishing, and the accomplishments you hoped for are coming to fruition. Your private plans are now public, and the hard work you've put in is paying off. It's a season of visibility and recognition, where your efforts are no longer just ideas but tangible achievements. This is the time to fully embrace growth, celebrate milestones, and continue pushing forward with confidence and purpose. In summer we feel seen, have peak energy levels, are celebrating and making an impact. We're in our lane, we've found a rhythm, and we're feeling confident. No wonder we don't want this season to end.

Autumn: The Season of Harvest and Reflection

In autumn we're just over the peak of the summer and are stepping back and reaping the rewards of our work. You've just moved into the house you've been renovating, sitting in your lounge, reflecting on the work that has gone on, enjoying what you have created. Other illustrations of life's autumn might be parenting teens, when the foundational work of the early years is bearing fruit but there's still careful guidance needed before they can step out as young adults. You might be reaching a point in your career where you've built a solid reputation and are seeing the results of years of effort, mentorship opportunities, and leadership roles, perhaps feeling a sense of mastery in your field.

It's a season of gratitude, reflecting on achievements, and stepping back to enjoy the view. But it's also a clear time of transition: something is coming to an end, and something new will be along soon. Things are changing, and you can sense it. You're basking in the last rays of the summer sun, but as the months of autumn pass by, you recognize that this time is now over. It's a bridging phase, and a necessary evaluation point. Autumn is a season of reflection, gratitude, and stewardship. It's a time to assess what has worked, to refine your direction, and to prepare for what's next. You might find yourself looking back with nostalgia, while also recognizing the inevitability of change. In this season, there's a sense of winding down from the intensity of summer, but it's not an ending just yet – it's a shift. This is also a time for consolidating lessons from the past and integrating them into your future. Autumn is beautiful, but it can also feel disconcerting. However, it is necessarily unsettling, preparing us for what's to follow.

Winter: The Season of Letting Go, Rest, and Renewal

Winter can be hard – bleak, even. Trees are bare, there are few signs of life, it's dark, it's cold, and it's challenging. Sometimes we find ourselves in winter seasons in our lives: none of us want them, and yet we know they must happen. To continue our house analogy, this would be the season when you're knocking the house down. There are no new foundations in place yet, just the hard work of dismantling and leaving the ground empty. What was known has now gone, and you can't yet see what's coming on the horizon. In life, winter might look like the end of a long-term relationship, where you're mourning what was and trying to imagine what life could be without it. It could be a time of grieving the loss of a loved one. Or it might be the loss of a job or a career path you've poured your energy into for years, leaving you feeling untethered and unsure of your identity. For some, it could be the empty nest years, when the children have moved out and the home that was once filled with noise and activity is now quiet and still. You can feel like spring is so far away, and all you're doing is letting go, missing out, and feeling forgotten. When you're in a winter, it seems like everyone else is in spring or summer. There's life and newness and celebration all around, but all you're doing is noticing what's missing and can't see what is coming next.

But it's not all doom and gloom. While winters can feel barren, they also hold immense potential. Beneath the surface, even when the ground looks empty, the soil is resting and preparing itself for new growth. It's a time to pause, reflect, and let go of what no longer serves you. Winters teach us resilience and the necessity of rest before renewal. They strip away distractions, forcing us to confront our inner selves and paving the way for the clarity and courage needed to start anew. If we lean into it, it can be a time of rest, reflection, and preparation as we ready ourselves for the coming spring. Spring happens only when winter has prepared the way.

Coaching Notes: Helen's Story

Helen came for coaching during a challenging season of her life. Initially, her goal was to explore her strengths and talents, using that self-awareness to guide her towards her next career step. At 39, Helen was deeply established in a legal career that she had poured countless hours, energy, and emotion into. But at the start of our coaching journey, she faced an unexpected loss – saying goodbye to her beloved dog, a loyal companion for many years. The grief hit her harder than she anticipated, and it seemed to open a deeper well of sadness she had avoided confronting.

It became clear that before we could focus on her future, Helen needed to address the present. She had to pause, reflect, and fully process her current reality. It was important for her to recognize the signs of the moment, reflect on them, and then determine her next steps. Through this process, Helen came to understand that she was in a winter season of life. She had recently experienced significant losses: the end of a relationship that had seemed to promise marriage, the painful realization that she hadn't yet become a parent at the age she had always expected, and the disappointment that a career she had invested so much into felt unfulfilling. Only once Helen processed the difficult emotions attached to this season could she begin to imagine what life might look like next. Along with therapeutic counselling to support our work together, we started to plan her next season, one step at a time.

As you read these descriptors of seasons, one may resonate deeply with where you are right now – you can spot the signs and know that's how life feels. For some, there may be a mix of seasons: one aspect of your life feels more like autumn, while another carries the hopes of spring. That's fine, and equally valid. The following reflection is designed to help orient you around where life is right now, not to box you into a single season or oversimplify your experience. Life is rarely one-dimensional, and recognizing the nuances of your journey can help you better navigate the opportunities and challenges of each area.

✎Activity: Identify Your Season

It's time to get out your journal and reflect on the season of your life right now. This is not the time to jump ahead to action, it is simply a moment to see the season for what it is, both the good and the bad. Use the prompts below to help guide and frame your thinking, but don't feel constrained by them.

- Which season of life do you feel most aligned with right now: spring, summer, autumn, or winter? Why? Or do you feel like different seasons apply to different parts of your life?
- Can you identify any recent events or shifts in your life that have caused you to feel like you're in a particular season? Can you describe them?
- What aspects of your current season are challenging for you, and what are the opportunities they present for growth or reflection?
- What part of you is being "rebuilt" or "renewed" in this season? What new opportunities or possibilities could emerge from the challenges you face right now?

Transition: It's Always Darkest Before the Dawn

You may feel caught between seasons, in those moments when one chapter ends and another is just beginning – like an endless autumn, perhaps. This is a time of transition, and these can be incredibly difficult.

Transition is the shift from one phase to the next, whether in action or a state of being. It's the *in-between moment*, when what was here has ended, but what is yet to come hasn't fully arrived. When I went into labour with my first child, I was fortunate to have an incredible midwife named Lisa. Our little boy had decided to make his entrance in the world sooner than expected, and everything happened quickly. I was progressing well, but there came a moment when I felt completely overwhelmed. I broke down in tears, convinced I couldn't go on. I felt so far from holding my baby, and so desperate. The pain was immense: I couldn't go back, but I couldn't see what lay ahead. I felt out of control. Lisa calmly explained that I was in what is known as "transition". This is the phase of labour that occurs between the first and second stages and is often considered the most challenging part. You can't go back, but moving forward feels impossible. It's disorienting, and the earlier positivity disappears, leaving you wondering how you'll ever make it through. "This is a good sign, though," said Lisa, "and means that Hannah is so much closer than she realizes." Sure enough, Noah was born quickly after. I was far closer to the finish line than the starting line – I just couldn't see it for myself.

Does this sound familiar? Your situation might be entirely different, but the emotions of transition remain the same. Can you recall times in your life when you stepped into something new, only for the initial optimism to fade into confusion or despair? When the early sunshine turned to fog, leaving you disorientated and wishing you'd never started? Maybe you began a new job, excited about the fresh opportunity, only to become overwhelmed by unfamiliar systems, with impostor syndrome creeping in as you questioned whether you were truly capable. Or perhaps you relocated for a dream role, but after the initial excitement found yourself struggling to adjust, missing the comfort of what you left behind. I want you to know that feelings of confusion, disappointment, self-doubt, and the urge to retreat to familiar ground are completely normal. Times of transition are necessary as we purposefully step towards our next season. If you're in a painful time of transition, heed Lisa's words: this is a good sign. Hold on. You're so much closer than you realize. It's always darkest before the dawn.

9-enders

Speaking of transitions, there's something intriguing that happens when we reach the "nine" of our decade. It represents another "seasonal shift" to consider as we reflect on the present and navigate times of transition. The years leading up to a new decade – ages 29, 39, and so on – are often marked by deep self-reflection, according to research.[1] These "What am I doing with my life?" years prompt many to engage in behaviours that reflect an ongoing or unfulfilled search for meaning. An audit of "the meaningfulness of life" takes place, even if subconsciously, and people tend to reach one of two conclusions: either they happily conclude that their lives are indeed meaningful, or they decide that their lives lack meaning in at least one important domain. If people feel their lives lack meaning, they usually take action. The data shows that during these ages, people are more likely to take on new challenges, such as running a marathon for the first time, but they're also when rates of infidelity and even suicide tend to rise.[2]

The "9 year" feels like a year-long season of transition, when you know something is coming to an end but haven't yet stepped fully into the new. Our responses to this season of reflection can either foster growth or lead us down a path that distances us from our true purpose. If you're in or approaching a "9 year", embrace it, recognizing that it's a natural time to reflect. However, make sure to channel that reflection into setting the scene for a successful next decade, rather than letting it hold you back. That said, these moments of deep self-questioning aren't limited to the "9 years". Life has a way of nudging us to reflect at various points, as we're learning in this chapter, through unexpected change, loss, personal milestones, or even an unexplained sense of restlessness. Whether or not you're at the end of a decade, these principles still apply: the key is to use these moments as opportunities for growth rather than allowing them to create confusion or stagnation.

✏Activity: Transition

Transitions can feel unsettling, like standing in a fog, unsure of what's ahead. But often, the moment we feel most lost is the sign that we're closer to a breakthrough than we realize. Take a moment to reflect on where you are in your journey. Take out your journal and use these reflective questions as prompts for your thoughts.

- What area of your life feels like it's in transition right now?
- Reflect on a time when you experienced a transition. How did you handle it? What feelings come up for you when you're in a transitional phase, especially when you can't clearly see what's ahead?

- How do you typically respond to uncertainty? Do you resist, rush ahead, or sit with the discomfort?
- If you're in or approaching a "9 year" in your life (such as 29, 39, 49, and so on), what reflections or realizations have started to emerge about your life so far?
- How do you feel about the progress you've made in your life? Are there areas where you feel fulfilled or areas that still feel incomplete?
- What emotions are surfacing for you in this moment?
- What are the core values, beliefs, or experiences that can help steady you through this shift?
- If you fully trusted that this transition was leading you somewhere meaningful, how would that change the way you see it?

Transitions may feel uncertain, but they are also full of possibility. You are closer than you think.

Understanding Your Now: A Deep Dive into Daily Life

As well as understanding the overarching season that we are in, we also need to focus on the everyday details of the here and now – the ins and outs of your life. As the renowned nature writer Annie Dillard said, "How we spend our days is how we spend our lives."[3] The details of how we spend our days are packed with data that can help us take stock, identify the current state of play, and pinpoint what needs to change. But where should we start? Simply saying, "reflect on your daily life" is too broad to be practical. Instead, we'll examine everyday life like it's a pie, dividing it into slices and working through each one with intention.

Activity: Life Pie

Your life is made up of many important elements that together create purpose. To understand what needs to change, you must first take a close look at your day-to-day life and get a clear picture of what's working well, what's going great, and what could use improvement. Make notes in your journal and, using the questions and prompts provided, reflect on each area and rate it on a scale of 1–10: 1 being completely unfulfilled or in need of significant change, and 10 being deeply satisfied and aligned with your sense of purpose. Then step back and consider the overall picture to see where you might want to adjust things to align more closely with your purpose. This will provide a great starting point for the work you're going to do throughout this book.

Step 1: Contribution and work

I've purposefully not called this "career" because, although for many of you that will be the focus here, there will be plenty who are not currently in paid employment, and as we've discussed, your career does not define living a purposeful life. You might be at home raising children, actively looking for work, retired, or dedicating time to volunteering or creative projects.

This section of the pie is about how we spend the majority of our time contributing to the world around us – whether that's through professional endeavours, caregiving, community involvement, or pursuing other projects and goals. While it could be about your career, please choose the definition of work that best suits your life stage right now. Whether you're in paid employment or not, it's worth noting that according to research, only 18 per cent of us believe that we get as much purpose from our work, whatever form it takes, as we would like to.[4] This is an opportunity to reflect on whether your contribution, work, and career feels fulfilling, purposeful, and sustainable, or whether adjustments are needed to better align with the life you want to lead.

- What does "work" mean for you right now?
- Think about a typical day in your life when you're engaged in your work or daily responsibilities. Which activities would you describe as "great", which ones feel "good", and which do you find to be "not so good"?
- Does your current work allow you to show up as your best self? In what ways does it support or hinder that?

Score this out of 10.

Step 2: Home and family

Your home life, whatever that may look like for you in this season, includes the time you spend in your home and the relationships you have with those closest to you. You might be navigating life as a parent or caregiver, managing the demands of a busy household, raising children, living alone, or supporting extended family in other ways.

This part of the pie is about how we invest our time in the home environment – whether that's caring for loved ones, nurturing relationships, managing daily household responsibilities, or creating a space that supports our wellbeing. It's an opportunity to reflect on whether your home and family life feels balanced, fulfilling, and aligned with your values, or if adjustments are needed to better support the life you want to build. For some, this area will go hand in hand with work outside the home, while for others it may serve as a primary or supporting focus of how time is allocated.

- Think about a typical day in your life right now when you're engaged in your home and family life. Which activities would you describe as "great", which ones feel "good", and which do you find to be "not so good"?
- Does your home life feel balanced, fulfilling, and aligned with the life you want to create?

Score this out of 10.

Step 3: Leisure and fun

This is about the time you spend enjoying yourself, unwinding, and engaging in activities that bring you joy. Leisure and fun aren't just about escaping from responsibility; they're essential for recharging, nurturing creativity, and maintaining a healthy work–life balance. Whether it's spending time on hobbies, exploring new interests, travelling, or simply relaxing, this part of your life plays a key role in your wellbeing. Reflecting on the time you dedicate to leisure and fun can reveal whether you're prioritizing joy and relaxation or if this aspect of your life has been crowded out by other commitments.

I am fully aware that for many of you reading this book, this area might be neglected. I was with a group of leaders recently, and when I asked what they did for leisure and fun, one busy working parent of little ones said "sleep". But, even when time is limited, it continues to be important for our sense of purpose and it needs our attention. It's an opportunity to assess whether you're making space for experiences that nourish your spirit and bring you happiness, and how these activities align with your values and sense of fulfilment.

- What do you do, in a typical week (or month if it's easier) for leisure and fun?
- Being realistic with your life stage, are you happy with the amount of time you give to it?

Score this out of 10.

Step 4: Friendship and connection

Consider the relationships and connections you have with others – whether through close friendships, social networks, or a sense of belonging to a broader community. Human connection is vital to our wellbeing, providing support, joy, and shared purpose. In fact, one study showed that participants' stress, happiness, and wellbeing levels were better predicted by their social circle strength than by the physical health data collected on a fitness tracker.[5] Whether it's spending time with friends, participating in social groups, or contributing to community initiatives, these connections help us feel grounded and valued.

On the flipside, loneliness can have a profound impact on our mental and physical health, reducing our sense of purpose.[6] On a personal note, I know that when I'm taking the time to stay connected to those that I love – investing in family, friends, and my community – life feels better, more balanced, and more purposeful, but it's so easy for it to be squeezed out of a busy schedule. Reflecting on your friendships and wider community involvement allows you to assess whether you feel connected and supported, or if there are areas where you could nurture deeper relationships or expand your social network.

- How would you describe your current social circle? Do you feel supported by your friends and community, or are there areas where you feel disconnected or isolated?
- What type of connection brings you the most joy and fulfilment?
- Do you feel a sense of belonging in any community or group?

Score this out of 10.

Step 5: Emotions and energy

Emotions are at the core of how we experience life, influencing our thoughts, behaviours, and relationships. Whether it's feelings of joy, stress, excitement, or overwhelm, our emotions are constant signals that can guide us towards a deeper understanding of ourselves. Obviously, a single emotion in isolation isn't necessarily a reflection of how your life is going. However, if you notice a recurring emotion or feeling, it's important to pay attention to the pattern.

Similarly, the energy we have – physical, mental, and emotional – plays a crucial role in how we navigate the demands of life. Are you feeling drained or energized by your daily activities? I know there are activities in my daily life that energize me, boost my mood, and make my routine feel more meaningful. In contrast, there are also plenty of things that drain my energy, emotionally exhaust me, and leave me questioning my direction. My energy levels and emotional state are important barometers for assessing the sense of purpose in my everyday life.

Reflecting on your emotional and energetic wellbeing gives you the opportunity to assess whether your emotional state is serving you, how you can better manage your energy levels, and whether your emotions align with the life you want to live. Understanding these aspects allows you to make more conscious choices about where to direct your energy, helping you feel more balanced and aligned with your true self.

- What emotions do you notice recurring in your daily life? Are there certain feelings (like joy, stress, frustration, or excitement) that come up frequently? What might these emotions be trying to tell you about your life right now?
- When you reflect on your energy levels, what stands out to you? Are there particular activities or people that energize you, while others leave you feeling drained? Make a list.

Score this out of 10.

Analyse your results

As you look at the five areas of your life pie, what do you notice? What scores are high, and which could do with some help? What's working and what isn't? What is giving you energy and what is draining it from you? What lifts your emotions and what doesn't?

What's missing? What do you need more of? Less of? What do you need to change? What themes are developing?

You Are Here

So, you have taken the time to properly assess your life right now. You've recognized the season of life you are in, spotted the signs of transition, and evaluated your day-to-day life in detail. Let's pull all this learning together and discover the key themes for you to build from.

- How has knowing the current season helped you feel more optimistic for the future?
- What season would you hope is coming next for you?
- What part of your life is in transition right now? What are you feeling about life on the other side of this shift, and what do you hope to gain or discover as you navigate through it?
- Reviewing your reflections from the Life Pie activity, which areas of your life feel most fulfilling, and which ones need more attention or adjustment?
- As demonstrated in the 1 in 60 rule of navigation, small deviations can lead to significant shifts over time. Are there any areas in your life where you sense you might be off course? What steps can you take to realign?
- If you could wave a magic wand and make one change in your life right now, what would you choose?

Key Takeaways

Understanding where you are in life is the essential first step in navigating where you want to go. Life, like the seasons, moves through phases of new beginnings, growth, reflection, and renewal, each offering unique lessons and opportunities for growth.

To make sense of your current season and chart your next steps:

- **Identify your season**: recognize whether you're in spring (new beginnings), summer (growth and momentum), autumn (reflection and preparation), or winter (letting go, rest, and renewal). Each season is valuable and necessary for a balanced life.
- **Embrace transitions**: transitions can feel disorienting as we let go of one thing and wait for the next, but they often signal that you're closer to a breakthrough than you think. Reflecting on these shifts can bring clarity and courage.
- **Take stock of your life**: use tools like the Life Pie to evaluate key areas – work, home, relationships, leisure, and emotional energy. Spot what's working, what's draining you, and where small adjustments can create meaningful change.
- **Remember the power of small steps**: like the 1 in 60 rule, even small course corrections can have a significant impact on your long-term direction. Reflecting and realigning ensures your journey is purposeful and fulfilling.

Clarity begins with self-awareness, and growth follows reflection. It's important to take the time to understand the present so that we can move forward into the future with purpose.

Chapter Two

The Guide

Identify Your True Strengths

I want to shift your thinking. I want you to be free from the constant pull of the world to fixate on what you are not, and instead to start focusing on all the wonderful things that you *are*. I want your perspective to transform from one that focuses on what you might lack to one that concentrates on your strengths. If this truth can become deeply rooted in your mind, heart, and actions, then you'll make significant progress on your journey towards a more purposeful life. I'd argue it's almost impossible to do so without it.

This curious counterintuitive instinct to fixate on our weaknesses seems hardwired into many of us. But this tendency, I believe, isn't inherent – it's shaped by the way the world works. Being constantly reminded of our shortcomings is not only the foundation of modern advertising but is also embedded in the culture of many organizations. Entire industries thrive on convincing us that we must be more, do more, and have more to feel like we are enough. We receive a school report and instinctively focus on the subject with the lowest grade. When we get feedback from our boss, even if most of it is glowing, we often forget the praise while the single area for improvement takes up permanent residence in our memories. We obsess over the "could do better" and "needs improvement" comments, while minimizing or even discounting the good and outstanding feedback that truly deserves our attention.

It can feel like the sensible thing to do: we need to work on what we don't do very well to grow, right? Well, no, not really.

You see, I hate to break it to you, but something that we're not designed to be, which doesn't engage our strengths, is never going to be a representation of us at our best. Something that doesn't come naturally, that we must work impossibly hard to improve – which we probably don't even enjoy – isn't going to give us life or light up those around us. It's just going to pull us away from living the life we were meant to be living. If it helps to make my point, let's take the focus off us mere mortals for a second and consider the greats. Imagine if Monet, the founder of Impressionism, had said, "Yes, I know I am rather good at painting, and I love the process of a piece of art coming to life, but I'm a rather average horse rider and so I need to spend much more of my week focusing on that." Or what if the world-renowned civil rights activist Martin Luther King Jr, based on improvement feedback, decided to work on his data analysis skills rather than spend his time perfecting his natural ability to communicate and deliver a compelling message? What a tragic waste of talent that would be. What might the world have missed out on if those were the decisions they had made, if they'd spent their days developing weaknesses into mediocrity rather than developing strengths into excellence?

What makes you any different from these examples? You have natural gifts, things that only you can do, and if you spend most of your time thinking about what you're not and what you can't do, then you will struggle to live a life of purpose and the world will miss out on who you really are. Think of it in a different way. If I assume that most readers of this book will be at least 20, that means, based on an average life, you have probably had a quarter of your life already. If you're nearer my age and have hit 40, you've had about half your allotted time here on Earth. Life is limited, and the hours we have at our disposal to develop ourselves are limited and rapidly ticking by; why would we choose to spend them trying to get better and be better at things we weren't even intended to do?

At the risk of sounding cheesy – I don't care, I'm going to do it – you are uniquely brilliant, designed to bring an inimitable set of talents to the world around you. It's time to wake up to your worth and start becoming a more magnificent version of who you were made to be.

The Strengths-Based Philosophy: It's Nothing New

Positive psychology, the area of psychology that the strengths-based approach sits in, began around the 1950s and only really gathered pace in the 1990s. But its roots stretch much further back than this. The phrase *Gnothi Seauton*, or "Know Thyself", was inscribed above the entrance to the Temple of Apollo in Delphi in ancient Greece, and the Greek philosopher Socrates developed the concept of truly knowing who we are as being the basis of wisdom and purpose around 2,400 years ago. About a hundred years later, Aristotle's concept of *eudaimonia* built on these foundations: one of those tricky to translate words, it centres on human flourishing and contentment – on having a "good soul". I love the idea of *eudaimonia* and think it's a concept for us to hold on to as we pursue our purpose. Aristotle maintained that true happiness comes from cultivating virtues, which are innate capacities or strengths like courage, wisdom, and temperance. He believed that everyone has unique capabilities, and that fulfilment comes from developing these personal strengths.

Many of the early faith writers built on this idea of knowing who we are and understanding that we each have special gifts to bring to the world, for the good of others and for our own sense of enjoyment and fulfilment.[1] But as time went by, these views based on understanding humans at their best became obscured by a fixation on human dysfunction. Somewhat understandably, the world of psychology developed a focus on what's going wrong, the reasons why we struggle, and human weaknesses. The attention was focused on what was missing. Pioneering psychiatrists like Sigmund Freud and Carl Jung centred their work around understanding suppressed memories, the subconscious, the unconscious mind, and the shadow self.[2] They used this work to understand dysfunction, disorder, neuroses, and inner conflicts.

Enter stage left the Positive Psychologists. In striking contrast to the philosophy of weakness fixing, they set about the topic of human wellbeing from a completely different starting place. First Dr Don Clifton and later Martin Seligman emphasized a need to identify and then maximize an individual's strengths to foster personal development and wellbeing. They firmly believed that weakness fixing would never lead to human flourishing, let alone *eudaemonia*. The point of their work was to demonstrate that we need to make our positive traits and talents the centre of our attention. We start with strengths: we work hard to discover exactly what they are, we practise and develop them, and this leads us to a purposeful life, a life that's good for us and leads us towards meaningful work.

Why Focusing on Strengths Works

If I've not yet convinced you that this approach makes sense, that it's the best use of your time here on Earth, then try this simple illustration. Pick up a pen or pencil and pop it in your non-dominant hand. Now write on a page, "I have unique strengths and talents". Do this 10 times.

How does it feel?

Granted, this doesn't work if you're ambidextrous, but for most of us, trying to work with our "wrong" hand is slow, poor quality, and downright frustrating. Some of us will dig in and the quality might improve a bit, but the majority will lose interest and the quality will be pretty shocking by the 10th iteration. Even if we do get better, it's a clunky and uncomfortable use of our time and energy. None of this is rocket science: focusing on what we do best will generate better and better results. Spending too much time on what we find hard might elicit some improvement if we're lucky, but it's highly unlikely to reach the standards our natural talents can reach. And it's likely to leave us dissatisfied, bore us to tears, or drive us to distraction.

Part of my work is with business owners and leaders, encouraging them to use this approach in their team and personal development. They love a bit of data, some hard facts as to why this works, and I get it: a fluffy feeling inside isn't always enough – we want to know the impact, the outcomes, and the reasons why we should do it. So let's look at some of that data together. A study that analysed over two million employees found that those that got to use their strengths and talents every day were six times more likely to be engaged in their jobs and three times more likely to report an excellent quality of life.[3] Engagement in our work is simply the measure of how we feel about what we do – and it's a pretty important metric if we want to live a life of purpose. If we're engaged, we're connected, committed, motivated, and aligned. Who wouldn't want to feel like this about work by simply doing the stuff we are made to do on the daily?

But there's more. I love this bit of research from Seligman and fellow psychologist Dr Tracy Steen. They enabled participants in their study to first get to know their signature strengths[4] and talents, then encouraged them to set about using them every day in a new or developed way. They wanted to see what impact it would have on their happiness, and/or depressive symptoms. They discovered that those that completed this task showed evidence of increased happiness and a decrease in depressive symptoms. The startling thing here is that the effects seemed to last up to six months, even though they'd only been asked to commit to the daily task for one week.[5] Now, they may well have continued to use their strengths like this by choice (and it seems many did), but this data gives us a significant key to living a life of purpose: discover your unique talent DNA and then put it to work every day.

I could go on. Developing research suggests links to improved academic performance when we are encouraged to focus on our talents,[6] and we're more inclined to make progress towards our goals if we do it in a way that's aligned with our personality and strengths.[7] We're also a lot less likely to make mistakes, and we're able to get a great deal more done.[8]

Coaching Notes: Lizzie's Story

When I first started working with Lizzie, her past few years had been full of challenges. She'd lost her mum, and she'd had a son after a few years of heartache and trying, only to find herself suffering from post-natal depletion and depression. She'd picked herself back up and built a business that worked well around the needs of her family, but it just wasn't fulfilling her in the way she'd hoped.

And now here she was, with her five-year-old son off to school, and she found herself on the edge of a new era, feeling a little lost. "Misaligned, somehow," to use her words. The circumstances of life, the bigger losses and little letting goes, had left Lizzie empty, lacking confidence, and unable to clearly see what to do next, yet knowing that something needed to change.

It's hard to know what to do next when you can't noticeably recognize who you are or what you've got to bring to the table. After Lizzie and I had spent some time working out where her life was at right now – the good, the bad, and ugly of it – we then turned our attention to rediscovering who she is and understanding her unique strengths: what she brings to every situation, what gives her energy, and what other people love about her. The stuff that made Lizzie, Lizzie. I loved watching this process take place. There was penny-drop moment after penny-drop moment as Lizzie reacquainted herself with who she was at her best and realized just how little of that she was getting to do daily. In her own words:

"When I stopped and really took the time to discover my strengths, it honestly changed my life. I realized that I'm a natural communicator and love to process with others, and yet I still need time alone to think deeply; that I have a deep desire to keep learning, keep being curious, and that being bored or staying stagnant is my kryptonite. And although I'm a deep thinker, I am a deep feeler. I sense my own emotions and feel them fully, and I can intuitively pick up on the feelings of others, too.

I realized that things I'd previously seen as negative about me were actually the very things that made me me – and I found myself beginning to see them as positives. So now I recognize that it's good that I like to talk, it's good that I like to learn and do new things, it's good that I feel what others feel, and that my feelings have weight and meaning. Knowing this gave me the intel I needed to start building a life that drew me closer to my purpose. I'm one hundred per cent clear on what I can offer. I know my unique strengths and how I bring them to the table. I understand what drives me and the values that I live by that direct my focus. I'm empowered to make this next season a better fit to who I am made to be."

I'd love you to have your own version of Lizzie's story. But before we can set to work on defining your unique strengths and purpose, we need a bit more understanding of this concept. What even *is* a strength? And how do we discover our own? Let's look at some key principles so that you can begin to uncover your core talents.

True Strengths Energize You, They Don't Deplete You

A surefire way to tell if we are doing the stuff that we were made to do is that we get energized by doing it. If it's a true strength, it will invigorate us and we find ourselves replenished by doing it. That's not to say we will have endless energy and never feel tired, of course not – but there's good tired and downright exhausted, don't you think?

I know that a couple of my true strengths lie in connecting with people and communicating insights. So, when I've been out doing a day's workshop, meeting new people, speaking and delivering content, I am energized by it. I feel alive, and I can tell that my internal batteries are being recharged by the kind of activity I have been doing.

This gives us another important clue to help us spot the moments when we're living out our true strengths and talents. We feel good, we feel energized, and we feel uplifted. The things we were doing filled up the tank and left us feeling satisfied. Bestselling author of motivational business books Marcus Buckingham puts it simply: "A strength is an activity that strengthens you."[9]

Just a note of caution here: there can be such a thing as too much of a good thing, so if I have a week or two when I get the balance wrong and I'm doing too much speaking and spending too much time with people, I need to tap out. The same will be true for you, too, in your area of talent and strength. Pause this thought – we'll come back to it later.

A true strength doesn't drain us: it fills us up. It brings energy, satisfaction, and a sense of being alive, even if it leaves us tired. It's the kind of tired that feels good, not exhausting.

Activity: The Diary Hack

Get out your diary – either a paper diary or electronic diary, both work. If you don't have a diary (wow, how are you managing?) then open the camera roll on your phone and use that as a memory jogger.

Step 1: Look back through your diary

It's absolutely fine to go far back in time if need be. Write down a few things you did that you really enjoyed. These can be things that gave you a sense of satisfaction or you felt energized by. Don't overthink this, you're simply looking for the things that you'd say yes to again. Look at this list. What were you doing? What activities were you involved in? What aspects of your personality were at work?

Step 2: Now look ahead

See what's coming up in the future (your camera roll obviously won't work for this one). What are you looking forward to? List some activities, meetings, and social engagements and see if you can spot any themes developing. What kinds of activities are a "definite yes" activity? Whenever I do this, the stuff that I am drawn to includes people, talking, coming up with ideas, making stuff happen, and getting things started.

Step 3: Analyse your findings

Two things to consider: this might not be easy, and you may find it hard to find fulfilling things. And don't be too hard on yourself, try to look for clues, for glimmers even. If it helps, it's fine if your examples come from time gone by and not just the current season. It doesn't have to be work activities – it all counts. Make a note of any patterns or themes that you can see developing.

If you want to take this idea further, you could always do the same activity and ask yourself the opposite question: what has drained you and what are you not looking forward to? For me, these would be activities that involve too much detail (I genuinely find myself feeling a bit sick when I have to get into the details) or trying to come up with ideas on my own. I learn from this that I am good at the big picture, and I'm better when collaborating. These things are also helpful clues – we learn what we are by also recognizing what we are not.

True Strengths Will Be Recognized by Others (Possibly Before You Do)

There's real power in other people's words, don't you think? You can probably think of many occasions when the words of others have bruised or deflated you. But what about the times when people's words have been spot on, recognizing our specific talent and praising us for it? Sadly, for many of us, those examples can often be counted on one hand (sidenote: we have got to get better at giving praise) but they are also keenly remembered and appreciated.

Now, there can be a bit of a problem. Sometimes people tell us what we bring, but we don't recognize it, or we play it down. If I had a pound for how many clients say to me, "But everybody does that, Hannah," I would be sipping a pina colada on a remote tropical island right now.

It's extremely common for people to minimize their unique strengths, feeling that their talents aren't particularly special and merely constitute being human. If you feel like that, please hear me when I say that things that come easily to you, that feel like "just being a decent person", don't come easily to everyone. If you're quick to see patterns in data and it all feels so obvious to you, please know that it's not obvious to the rest of us. If you're someone who strikes up conversations with anyone and everyone, enabling that person to feel included and liked, then please hear that this is a gift that we don't all possess. If you're someone who sees the future clearly, or understands how the past impacts the present, if you're flexible, if you're ordered, if you're innovative, if you're detailed – all these things may feel normal, or average, or easy for you, but they aren't for us all. So, when you receive feedback, if people notice things about you, take note of it. Literally write it down somewhere. And then think of these comments like clues, breadcrumbs on the path, guiding you towards a deeper understanding of who you are and why that matters.

True strengths are often seen more clearly by others than by ourselves. What feels ordinary to us – our natural abilities – can be exceptional to those around us. Listen to their words; they hold inklings to the gifts that make us unique.

✎Activity: What Three Words

I'd love you to be brave and gather yourself some feedback that helps to sharpen your understanding of yourself. Get in touch with a handful of people – a friend, a loved one, a colleague, a family member, anyone you like – and ask them to describe you using only three positive words. Compile the list and see if you can identify any themes developing. Are there any surprises in there? Anything you just can't see? If so, be even braver and ask them to tell you more about what this looks like to them. You just might start to see it in yourself, too.

True Strengths Stand the Test of Time

Often, when people discover more about their strengths and talents, their response to me is, "Well, I do that because I am an accountant/doctor/[insert current job]." But this can't be the whole truth, because if it was, it would suggest that every accountant/doctor/[insert any profession you like] was a carbon copy of the rest of them, and we all know this isn't the case. I know from personal experience of working with thousands of professionals that there is no one type or set personality for any of the roles I've encountered. Of course, certain innate talents are potentially advantageous for particular roles. However, not only are these talents not role-related, but your talents also predate your role. They are much more of a reflection of who you are than your current life scenario and job title.

There's so much discussion around the nature versus nurture debate. Are we who we are because it's our innate personality and DNA, or are we a product of our experiences? The problem is, we can't extricate ourselves from our childhood or our genetics, so we're never going to get a definitive answer. But research does give us some guidance. First, we can gather some clues from studies into the lives of twins. In one study that compiled the findings of over 50 years of classical twin studies (which compared the similarity of traits between identical twins and fraternal twins to determine the influence of genetics versus environment), they concluded that we inherit about 50 per cent of our make-up.[10]

Additionally, in a study spanning four decades, researchers examined how personality traits from childhood aligned with adult behaviour. In the 1960s, elementary school teachers rated the personalities of children in a long-term research project called the Hawaii Personality and Health Cohort. Forty years later, these individuals were interviewed on video in a clinic. Coders reviewed these recordings to assess behaviours. Traits like verbal fluency in their childhood linked to social confidence in adulthood; children that scored high adaptability corresponded with cheerfulness and curiosity; early impulsivity related to later talkativeness; and self-minimization was tied to humility and insecurity further down the line.[11]

We can grow, yes, but do we change? Maybe not so much. And this is no bad thing.

I look at my own children, now teenagers and young adults. My eldest son was always focused, responsible, and loyal. He still is. My middle boy was always adaptable, perceptive, and brilliant at meeting new people. Still sounds like him. My youngest son was always quick-witted, confident, and goes at one hundred miles an hour. He's showing no signs of changing.

Are they growing? Yes.

Are they changing? I'm not so sure.

True talents aren't defined by our roles: they are reflections of who we are, rooted long before any job title. We may grow and adapt, but our core traits often remain surprisingly constant.

Activity: Flip the School Report

Let's take some feedback from time gone by and see if it can give clues as to our true strengths and talents. Do you remember your school report? If you're anything like me, you can remember some of the more brutal bits. Here's a couple of direct quotes from mine:

"She is aware of how much she could improve her concentration by quietening her mind and tongue!"

"As with her classwork, Hannah's examination paper showed a lot of carelessness. Hannah must learn to settle and not shout out, realizing that there are 30 other children to be taught."

"She must make sure she doesn't let her enthusiasm bubble over into distractedness."

These are selected highlights (well, lowlights), and they did say some nice things too (some of them). I would, however, like to say that there was definite room for improvement when it came to encouragement from my teachers, as well as room for improvement from me.

Examine your own feedback

I want you to take some of your own undesirable feedback and consider the following. What is the positive spin on the negative school report? If you can't remember the school report, what other negative feedback have you received that's got a strength lurking inside it, if you could just give it some fine tuning? Make a list of a few comments you've heard over the years and try to see them in a new, improved light.

For example, "too chatty" becomes "excellent communicator"; "away with the fairies" turns into "innovative thinker"; "distracted" now reads as "multitasker".

Important note: putting a positive spin on my feedback doesn't make it any less true. It doesn't mean I wasn't too chatty or too distracted. It was a strength in a raw form, that without mature application just came across as too much. I'm learning to use these talents much more positively, year after year. Now I can say I'm a keen communicator and able to juggle with the best of them.

True Strengths Are More Than What You Can Do – They're What You Want to Do

The first thing to realize, when we're talking about discovering true strengths and talents, is that it is so much more than just writing a list of what you can do. In fact, that's not always particularly useful, because there's plenty of things we have *learnt* to do that we don't *love* to do. For example, I am a fairly organized person, and most of my friends would say I'm one of the more organized among us, but this isn't something that I would say comes naturally to me and nor is it something I really love. I know people who are way better at this than I am, and for them it is a thing of joy – creating order from chaos and putting everything in its place. Part of me would love for this to be one of my natural strengths, but really it's a learnt one.

We must be careful to distinguish between the things we have learnt to do, which we've perhaps even become pretty good at, and the things we would choose to do and are drawn towards. The latter are more instinctive, and they are our natural preferences, regardless of obligations and learnt behaviours. I've heard it described as the magnetism of the body – a pull that we can't always explain, it's just who we are.

True strengths aren't just things we've learnt to do well – they're the things that naturally draw us in, that we'd choose again and again. While skill can be developed, true talent feels like second nature.

There are some brilliant tools out there that you could choose to use. The one that I like the most is the CliftonStrengths®, whose accuracy and specificity I love. There's also the Enneagram, Myers-Briggs Type Indicator®(MBTI), VIA® Character Strengths, DiSC®, and the Big Five®, to name a few more. All these kinds of personality assessments help us to build a picture of who we are and how we tick. You can, however, begin to discover your true strengths by using the principles and activities in this chapter, in conjunction with the simple "strength types" activity I've created to help you get more specific about who you are at your best.

Activity: Strength Types

I've spent the last decade of my career focusing on personality, talent, strengths, and purpose, and I have taken those experiences and designed a simple framework to help you discover your true strengths. This is something that you can use right here and now, to accompany your processing throughout this book. Drawing on my learning, I've defined eight personality characteristics that cover various key strengths. But before I give you the descriptors of the eight different types, I want you to answer some questions to help you assess yourself.

Give yourself a score from 0–7 for how much each statement resonates with you, 0 being nothing like you and 7 being absolutely you. Be honest! This is not about who you'd like to be or who you think sounds more impressive, it's about who you actually are. Add up your scores and see which of the types resonate most strongly with you.

Type A	0	1	2	3	4	5	6	7
I feel most accomplished when I set specific goals and see them through to completion								
I enjoy tackling tasks in an organized, step-by-step manner to ensure they're done efficiently								
When I commit to a project, I am driven to overcome obstacles and make steady progress								
Consistency in my approach is important to me; I enjoy creating and sticking to routines								
Total Score:								

Type B	0	1	2	3	4	5	6	7
I often find myself analysing situations to uncover patterns or underlying causes								
I enjoy thinking about long-term strategies and making detailed plans for the future								
I frequently come up with innovative ideas and look for new ways to solve problems								
I enjoy gathering facts and examples to help inform current decisions								
Total Score:								

Type C	0	1	2	3	4	5	6	7
I am naturally attuned to the emotions of those around me and strive to support them								
Building meaningful, authentic relationships is important to me								
I feel a sense of fulfilment when I can help bring people together and foster a positive atmosphere								
I feel a sense of satisfaction when I can create harmony and support among people								
Total Score:								

Type D	0	1	2	3	4	5	6	7
I am energized by opportunities to influence others and lead them towards a common goal								
I enjoy persuading others and feel comfortable sharing my ideas with a group								
I feel confident taking charge in situations and making decisions, even when others may be uncertain								
I enjoy opportunities to share my thoughts and inspire others to take action								
Total Score:								

Type E	0	1	2	3	4	5	6	7
I often reflect on my life's purpose and seek meaning in my actions								
I feel a strong sense of duty to follow through on my commitments and take ownership of my actions								
I make decisions that align with my core values and sense of purpose								
I find meaning in being part of something larger than myself, feeling connected to a purpose or cause that extends beyond my personal goals								
Total Score:								

Type F	0	1	2	3	4	5	6	7
I am curious and love discovering new ideas, skills, or areas of knowledge								
I am excited by new experiences and embrace opportunities for personal growth								
I am adaptable and enjoy exploring different approaches to familiar challenges								
I thrive in situations where I can adapt to new circumstances and find creative solutions to unexpected challenges								
Total Score:								

Write down the types as you scored in rank order. What are your top three types?

Understanding the Personality Types

Now that you know your scores, let me give you some definitions for each of the personality types. Remember, these are broad definitions, and you won't agree with it all. Just take the good stuff and start to assimilate it as the strength within you.

Type A: The Achiever

You get stuff done, you execute, you produce results, and you thrive on that satisfying feeling of completion. To-do lists? You love them, and you probably have one for the weekends, too. You feel most accomplished when you set specific goals and see them through to completion. Whether it's a work project or a personal challenge, you tackle tasks with an organized, step-by-step approach, ensuring everything is done efficiently. When you commit to something, nothing can stand in your way; your drive to overcome obstacles keeps you steadily progressing.

Type B: The Thinker

You're a natural problem-solver, always diving deep into ideas and concepts. You often find yourself analysing situations to uncover patterns and underlying causes, making sense of complexities in your world. If there's something not right, you're happy to lift the metaphorical bonnet and have a good diagnose. Thinking about long-term strategies excites you and you love making detailed plans for the future. You frequently come up with innovative ideas and seek new ways to tackle old challenges. Plus, you enjoy gathering facts and examples to inform your decisions, ensuring that your choices are backed by solid information.

Type C: The Connector

Building relationships is your forte, and you are naturally attuned to the emotions of those around you. You love to support others and create meaningful, authentic connections that enrich your life and theirs. You feel a deep sense of fulfilment when you can help bring people together and create a positive atmosphere, making everyone feel valued and included. Creating peaceful relationships with others brings you satisfaction, and you thrive in environments where collaboration and mutual support flourish. Your empathetic nature allows you to connect on a deeper level, making you a trusted friend and collaborator.

Type D: The Impactor

You have a magnetic presence that energizes those around you, and you thrive on opportunities to influence others and lead them towards a common goal. You enjoy persuading people and feel comfortable sharing your ideas with a group, sparking engaging conversations that inspire action. Confidence comes naturally to you, especially when taking charge in uncertain situations; you're not afraid to make decisions and guide others. You look forward to the chance to share your thoughts, motivating and inspiring those around you to embrace change and pursue their aspirations. Your enthusiasm spreads through the group, making you a powerful force for positive impact.

Type E: The Believer

You often find yourself reflecting on your life's purpose, seeking meaning in your actions and the choices you make. It's got to matter for it to be worth it. A strong sense of duty drives you to follow through on your commitments and take ownership of your decisions. You're guided by your core values, making choices that resonate with your sense of purpose. You find fulfilment in being part of something larger than yourself, feeling connected to a cause or mission that extends beyond your personal goals. Your authenticity shines through as you strive to align your actions with what truly matters to you, creating a life rich in meaning and significance.

Type F: The Explorer

Adventure is your middle name. You're naturally curious and love discovering new ideas, skills, or areas of knowledge. New experiences excite you and you eagerly embrace opportunities for personal growth, always looking for ways to expand your horizons. Adaptability is one of your strong suits, as you enjoy exploring different approaches to familiar challenges. You thrive in situations where you can navigate new circumstances and find creative solutions to unexpected problems, making life a never-ending adventure, full of possibilities. Your open-mindedness and willingness to explore the unknown lead you to exciting discoveries every day.

Coaching Notes: Ben's Story

Ben came to work with me after redundancy left him wondering what might be next. He'd experienced quite a hurtful departure from his previous place of work, and his confidence was at rock bottom. He felt misunderstood, misrepresented, and lost. He had given a lot to his last employer and genuinely believed in what they stood for. Now here he was, in the middle years of life, looking for his next assignment while trying to restore his self-esteem.

As we worked together on discovering his true strengths, Ben realized he had dismissed so much of his personality as being role-related, because he had a certain job that necessitated that skill. He started to realize the "why" underneath it all – why he did the things he did, why he led the way he led, and some of the reasons why he was feeling the way he was about leaving his previous role.

"As I began to rediscover my talents and learn to appreciate my personality, I stopped taking things for granted. I recognized that what I contribute doesn't come naturally to everyone, and that as I look ahead to my next role, this is the way I need to represent myself – no longer seeing myself as a generic or cookie-cutter leader, but more able to say the things that I do well, the things that give me energy and life, and the things that others appreciate about me.

I now realize that my values-driven approach is part of my DNA, that I am led by my core beliefs, which means that I take what I am doing seriously, wanting to not just get the job done but to do it to the best of my ability. I know now that I am an analytical thinker, ready to question, look for patterns, and diagnose the problem using logic. I love metrics and measures; they motivate me to work hard and there's nothing better for me than meeting a challenging goal I believe in. When I began this process, I never expected to be able to talk about myself with such clarity and conviction. I couldn't really see or appreciate who I am, but now I know what I bring and what I need in order to thrive."

I'm hoping the learning and reflective activities within this chapter are beginning to shift your thinking – moving you from a deficit or scarcity mindset to a strengths-based abundance mindset. There's a place for understanding our weaknesses (it happens to be Chapter 5), but the focus of our minds and our time should be on looking at what we have and growing that into something special. There are talents that you possess that you are minimizing and overlooking. There are gifts that you bring to the world that until now you haven't realized don't come easily to others. There are strengths within you that right now you may even see as a weakness. It's time to stop looking at what you're not and to start looking at what and who you are. With this fresh perspective, view your newly found strengths like an acorn in your hand: it doesn't look like much, and you could easily just throw it away, but it contains the kernel of so much promise and possibility.

Take your true strengths and plant them in your thoughts. Give them the conditions they need to thrive, nurture signs of growth, and protect them from their vulnerabilities.

Mighty oaks from little acorns grow.

Key Takeaways

Your natural strengths define you more meaningfully than your weaknesses. They tell you so much more about your personal purpose than a focus on what you're not ever could. Fixating on weaknesses is a distraction that limits potential, while building on strengths gives endless opportunity for development and fulfilment. When we live according to our strengths, we're happier, more productive, and improve our wellbeing.

True strengths have four key traits that give us clues to recognizing them:

- **True strengths energize rather than deplete:** they fill up your reserves and feel good (you can do too much of a good thing, though, so watch out for that)

- **True strengths will be recognized by others:** often even before you notice them yourself
- **True strengths stand the test of time:** they're evident in both your personality and behaviours from a young age, growing and developing rather than completely transforming into something else
- **True strengths reflect what you want to do, not just what you can do:** they are activities you naturally gravitate towards

To discover and then build on your true strengths:

- Reflect on activities that energize and excite you
- Gather feedback from people who know you well
- Take previous negative feedback and turn it on its head to create a positive in the making

To sum up, it's time to shed the scarcity mindset, embrace a strengths-based view, and nurture your innate talents to bring out your best.

Chapter Three

The Waterfall

Uncover What Makes You Unique

I've got a friend called Mads who has an interesting tattoo. It's of a word that I imagine most of us won't have heard before. That word is *poíēma* (pronounced poy-ay-mah). The short explanation is it's the ancient Greek word for poem. "But it's so much more than that," Mads explained. "It speaks to me of who I really am."

This is one of those untranslatable words that can still resonate deeply. Its meaning is discussed in early philosophy and features in sacred texts.[1] If we take the time to dig deeper, *poíēma* leans into the idea of something that has been crafted, a work of art, something matchless and divinely created. It hints at something that can perhaps only be fully understood and known by the creator. A one-off. A magnum opus.

For Mads it's a reminder of who she is: she's the human equivalent of a Rembrandt, crafted as a one-of-a-kind masterpiece. Tattooed on her arm is a reminder that she has been distinctively, divinely designed. She has a one-off role to play. A unique purpose to pursue. She's imperfectly perfect. She doesn't want to live as a pale imitation of herself or anyone else.

The same is true of you.

Let me give you a different way of looking at it. There's a documentary about the year-long process of crafting a Steinway, an instrument by the world's premier piano company. The method is defined by individuality and striving for perfection, from sourcing the Sitka spruce wood from Alaska to the meticulous attention to technique as the body is shaped, to the final details as the piano is completed. What's even more interesting is the fact that each Steinway piano is portrayed as having a distinct character, like none that have come before or will be made after. Wally Boot, a former final tone inspector at Steinway & Sons, explained: "I have pianos that have a different personality, on account of the wood and the hammer and the felt. Everything's handmade, so every piano is a little different and sounds a little different. Every piano's got its own personality, and we've just got to bring it out."[2]

Steinway pianos, snowflakes, fingerprints, cloud formations, iris patterns, DNA, auroras, tree rings, raindrops, moments in time, human beings: all unrepeatable phenomena.

Understanding Your Unique Design

Now we've waxed lyrical about the wonderfulness of you, let's get a little more practical. Why does this matter? First, it matters because of how you see yourself. On the surface you could write this off as unnecessary fluffy talk, but, like Mads, we all need reminding that we are a limited edition. Each of us carries a unique blend of strengths, experiences, and perspectives that no one else can replicate.

When we know who we uniquely are and how this feeds into our sense of purpose, it has a positive effect on our self-confidence. It becomes more than just self-awareness – it's self-assurance. We stop second-guessing our place in the room, our worth in conversations, and our value in the roles we play. Instead, we carry ourselves with a quiet confidence rooted not in external validation, but in an internal knowing. And when we have that level of clarity, it affects how we show up and how we speak about ourselves. We get to be who we are with deeper conviction and greater enjoyment, and a lightness comes from not trying to be someone we're not. For example, when you're in a team meeting and you know you're deep-thinking and curious, you take the time to form your thoughts and ask the best questions with assurance, rather than rushing to fill silence or prove yourself. When you're with a crowd of people and you know you're a funny storyteller, you embrace the moment, sharing your latest escapade with great aplomb, confident in your ability to bring joy to the room. When sitting in the interview chair, and you know exactly who you are, you move past platitudes and instead speak with originality and conviction, leaving an impression that feels both authentic and memorable. Each time you contribute your unique self you're living out your purpose.

Second, when we understand our unique design, it means we speak clearly and precisely about who we are, so others can see our worth. We start to show up in a way that means those around us get to identify, experience, and benefit from our unique contribution. When we stop apologizing, over-compensating, and/or minimizing and instead lean into who we have been made to be, our unique characteristics can begin to shine through and be recognized by others, too. This shift isn't just about external recognition; it's also about internal alignment. When we embrace our design, we stop wasting energy trying to fit into roles or expectations that were never meant for us. We can't keep expecting others to work out our worth for themselves, we need to help them get there through our words, actions, and decisions. This might look like advocating for ourselves in conversations, sharing our successes without downplaying them, or simply showing up consistently as our authentic selves. Over time, this clarity creates a ripple effect. Others start to trust us more, rely on us more, and value us more – not because we've demanded it, but because we've demonstrated it. Understanding and expressing our unique design isn't a one-time act; it's an ongoing commitment to showing up fully, courageously, and unapologetically as ourselves.

Finally, when we are at ease with our unique contribution, we can help others see who *they* are, too. Secure people enable others to feel secure. When we operate from a place of confidence in our own value, we create an atmosphere where others feel safe to explore, express, and embrace their own strengths without fear of judgement or competition. Firm in the knowledge of who you are, you can comfortably make space for others to be who they are, at no cost to your own security. There's no sense of scarcity – no need to compare, compete, or overshadow – because you understand that your worth isn't diminished by someone else's success. Instead, you become a catalyst for growth in others, encouraging them to lean into their strengths, discover their unique contributions, and show up authentically. You know what you uniquely do, and so nobody else can take that place. This isn't about being irreplaceable in an egotistical sense, but about recognizing that the specific blend of strengths, experiences, and perspectives you bring to the table is unique. In that understanding, you naturally create space for others to step confidently into their own roles without feeling the need to mimic or compete with you. When you model this kind of ease and assurance, you give others permission to do the same. It's a powerful cycle: your security fosters their security, and their growth amplifies your own. By being unapologetically yourself, you become a mirror for others to see their own strengths more clearly.

Reversing the Looking-Glass Self

In the digital age, where we're constantly bombarded by the opinions and influences of others, it can be difficult to look inwards and truly identify who we are at our core. There's a theory in social psychology termed The Looking-Glass Self. It was coined by Charles Horton Cooley in 1902 to describe how people form their self-concept based on their understanding of how others perceive them.[3] It argues that identity, self-esteem, and confidence are formed, and reformed, based on the perceptions of others. There are three steps in the process: a person in a social setting imagines how they appear to others, then that person imagines other people's judgement of that appearance, then they develop feelings about and respond to those perceived judgements.

Let me give you an example. You're going somewhere where there are going to be people you don't know, such as a networking event or a party. You imagine yourself to be funny, kind, and warm. When you're at the party, if the people smile at you, touch your arm, and perhaps laugh at your jokes then your opinion is confirmed. But if they seem disinterested, look away, leave the conversation, or pull back you might start to question your original beliefs. Of course, this theory is difficult to disagree with, as most of us form opinions of ourselves based on this kind of feedback. I know I do it: when I'm leading sessions and speaking at events,

I look for clues to see if what I have imagined is true and I update my perceptions accordingly. But there are problems with this behaviour. What if we get conflicting feedback? What if we misinterpret feedback? Furthermore, back in Cooley's day there wasn't social media, so the amount of feedback from social settings was reasonably limited. Now we are bombarded with feedback, so the scale of the perceptions and opinions to filter through is exhausting. I'm not even talking about the opportunity for comparison (we'll come to that later, my friend).

So, although the looking-glass self is central to our self-understanding (nobody wants to be a sociopath), should it be the primary way we decide who we are? Should it be the only way? I want to suggest that although the perceptions of others are vitally important (we will also come to this later), I don't want you to form who you are on that basis. Let it inform, guide, and nurture you, but don't let it define you. Turn that looking glass on yourself for a bit. Give yourself the job of uncovering your distinctive personality. Your perceptions matter, too.

Embrace Your Unique Self

I feel like I am spending an increasing amount of time online proving that I am, in fact, a human. You know those little tests that we have to do to show we aren't a bot? Things like looking at a squiggly set of numbers or words and having to decipher them, or clicking on all the boxes that have a motorcycle in them? These tests are called CAPTCHAS. I thought it was a play on the word capture and it's capturing my real identity or my sanity or something, but it's actually an acronym. It stands for "Completely Automated Public Turing Test to Tell Computers and Humans Apart".[4] And although this may sound like the biggest digression from a book about discovering purpose, I promise you, it isn't. I believe knowing the difference between humans and robots, on a much deeper level than whether we can pass certain random tests, is truly important. What differentiates us from an automated replacement will be increasingly significant as technology marches on. This is because there are skills and abilities we have that AI can also perform. However, it's not what you do, it's the way that you do it. Crucially, knowing the *way* you do stuff, the *way* you think, and the *way* you feel will not only distinguish you from a robotic alternative, but it will also give you the confidence to know how you stand out from other people and the reason why you make a difference.

One of the biggest issues that holds people back from truly embracing the uniqueness of who they are is the fear of being "too much". This phrase is one that reverberates around our heads, causing a spiral of overthinking and self-consciousness. There have been countless times when I've got in my car and driven away from an event or work situation and started to ruminate over whether I was "too much" in that environment. What did people really think of me? Was I too chatty, too enthusiastic, too passionate, too emotional, too opinionated? Possibly, at times, I was. But if I spend my life moderating my personality out of a fear of being too much, I'll end up contorting myself into someone who I am not. Ultimately, this isn't good for me, creating a dissonance inside that will negatively impact my wellbeing. And it's not good for those around me, either, because it means my bit of the jigsaw ends up being missing from the puzzle.

Now, I hope it's obvious that I am not saying we should ignore feedback, mindlessly dominate spaces, and refuse to grow. None of us are perfect (I'm definitely not, anyway), and taking on healthy criticism is often a very good reason to adjust, adapt, and mature. But if I am diminishing myself because I am worried about being too much, I'm behaving in a way that's rooted in fear, which isn't the best foundation for healthy growth.

Coaching Notes: Emma's Story

Emma came to me for coaching when she was beginning to feel like she had lost her sense of who she was. She said that work had become "everything", sucking the life out of her. On top of this, she felt like she wasn't being her true self in any setting: too tired for home and friendships and too toned down at work for fear of sticking out like a sore thumb in an environment where most of her colleagues felt different to her. But, in the middle of all this stretching and masking, there was one aspect of her role that she did especially love. That was her work with students and early-career professionals, teaching and mentoring them and watching them grow. She longed to do more of this, but worried that the decision makers would want someone less like her, someone less chatty and less enthusiastic by nature. When in meetings with other leaders, she could sense the difference between them, and rather than that being a good thing, it made her shrink who she was. She saw herself as the odd one out and so tried to fit in, be less enthusiastic, less communicative, less Emma.

As you can imagine, none of this worked out well for anyone, and so Emma finally decided to make some changes. When we started to work together, we first needed to reacquaint Emma with herself and then help her to see that self as a much-needed thread in the fabric of her team, family, and friendships. Once she had a better idea of who she was, as a starting place for growth I suggested she begin being 10 per cent more Emma in every environment.

"I could feel my confidence starting to return," she told me. "I began to recognize that hiding my strengths and talents rather than leading from this place was knocking my self-esteem and taking all the enjoyment out of work, and life, too." Fast forward a few months and I received the best message from Emma:

"You'll be pleased to know I've just been successful in an interview to double my education role from one day to two and that I unashamedly talked all about my ability to engage with anyone, connect with strangers, show empathy, communicate clearly, and bring a positive approach to the development of others. Thanks for giving me the courage to be, as you suggested, 'at least 10 per cent more me' – I think I was maybe more like 100 per cent though!"

Emma's story had a brilliant outcome for her and the people that love her. Leaning unapologetically into her unique design, she succeeded in getting to do more of what she loves. What would it feel like for you to be 10 per cent more you, in every environment? Grab a drink, a pen, and a notebook, and let's start to think about that in a little more detail.

✎Activity: True Strengths in High Definition

In the previous chapter, one of the activities gave you the chance to discover your particular strength type. Here, we're going to take that basic headline and give it some colour and definition.

Step 1: Identify

Write down your strength type (for example, the Achiever).

Step 2: Describe

Look at the description given in the previous chapter and note the bits that particularly resonate with you. Not all of it will, and that's okay (we are trying to move away from the generic and get more specific). Make a list of some key descriptive words or phrases that stand out to you.

Step 3: Analyse

Now, using the list of words on pages 80-81 as inspiration, choose some words that especially characterize the *way* in which you display this strength type.

Step 4: Define

Take your favourites from steps 2 and 3, and make a sentence like this: I am a .... achiever who ....

An example might be, "I am an organized achiever who takes my responsibilities seriously."

Step 5: Repeat

Repeat this for your top three strength types. This might look like:

"I am an organized achiever who takes my responsibilities seriously. I am an authentic believer who works best when I feel connected to a project that is bigger than me. I am an enthusiastic impactor who thrives in uncertain situations that need courage."

Step 6: Revise

You might want to take this work a little further, mixing and matching to show the interconnectivity between these traits and talents. Feel free to work and rework, tweaking and adding detail as you go. The more specifics you include, the better. So, you could end up with something more like this:

"I am an enthusiastic achiever who thrives in uncertain situations that need courage. I am an organized believer who takes my responsibilities seriously. I am an authentic impactor who works best when I feel connected to a project that is bigger than me."

Here are some words to help you get started with this activity. Please note this list is not exhaustive – feel free to use your own or dig into a thesaurus for more inspiration. The idea is to help you get more specific and double-down on your uniqueness. Not all of the words need apply to you.

Achiever

Organized • Efficient • Productive • Goal-focused • Committed • Process-driven • Resilient • Flexible • Adaptable • Predictable • Focused • Multi-tasker • Solo-performer • Team-orientated • Driven • Collaborative • Reliable • Responsible • Deliberative • Initiating • Consistent

Thinker

Future-focused • Contextual • Flexible • Creative • Imaginative • Innovative • Data-driven • Analytical • Problem-solver • Strategic • Detailed • Diagnostic • Deep • Mindful • Observant • Reflective • Considered • Quick • Pragmatic • Big-picture • Conceptual • Critical • Visionary

Connector

Empathetic • Deep • Warm • Open • Inclusive • Discerning • Harmonious • Compassionate • Supportive • Trustworthy • Understanding • Genuine • Kind • Intuitive • Insightful • Selective • Collaborative • Caring • Respectful • Honest • Encouraging • Friendly • Generous • Thoughtful • Perceptive

Impactor

Charismatic • Enthusiastic • Positive • Engaging • Communicative • Commanding • Confident • Inspirational • Motivating • Encouraging • Self-assured • Risk-taker • Magnetic • Influential • Bold • Empowering • Passionate • Articulate • Courageous • Proactive • Resilient

Believer

Purposeful • Authentic • Responsible • Grounded • Loyal • Reflective • Faithful • Ethical • Principled • Conscientious • Mindful • Connected • Faithful • Values-led • Purpose-driven • Mission-orientated • Steadfast • Ethical • Dutiful • Aligned • Dedicated • Serving • Committed

Explorer
Curious • Open • Growth-mindset • Knowledgeable • Open-minded • Adventurous • Visionary • Adaptable • Fearless • Tireless • Creative • Insightful • Inquisitive • Dynamic • Imaginative • Studious • Eager • Perceptive • Self-motivated • Growth-orientated • Perceptive

Tell Your Story

You've now delved deeper into your true strengths and talents and given yourself some specific language to help describe more clearly who you are. This is going to be brilliant for your confidence, your decision making, and to act as a signpost to those around you. Use it in interviews, conversations, and when you're trying to make yourself understood. This is great progress in our pursuit of purpose, but this isn't the whole picture by any means. There's something else that often gets missed at this point. We get focused on our strengths, talents, and personality and miss out a very important part of who we are. I believe this next step is vital: too many people that I work with have overlooked this completely and then been blindsided when starting out, returning to work, or choosing to do something different.

It's *your* story. Skills can be learnt, experiences can be gained, and even some talents are matched by others. But nobody has your story. It's uniquely yours, and it's shaped you in ways you may not even fully realize. Your past, your challenges, and your triumphs are all strands that have woven together to create the person you are today. We are all shaped by our experiences, and without acknowledging our unique stories we cannot truly understand who we are. The power of your story lies in its ability to guide you, to inform your choices, and to help you navigate your future. Let's dig into this some more, because by embracing your personal narrative, you'll uncover insights that will help you grow even further.

The Power of Your Story

In a coaching conversation recently, a client asked me to tell her my story. How did I get here, doing what I was doing? What were the events that led up to this work? Did I have a master plan that I had executed? I checked she was sure she wanted to use the session time to do this, and proceeded to tell her an abridged version of my life story. It included a bit about the work I'd done, some of the happier life events that had shaped my decisions (the big ones like love and children), and some of the more difficult moments that had also deeply impacted my life's direction.

It had quite an effect on us both. For her, it gave her confidence that ordinary people who put their unique strengths and talents to good use can do wonderful things. Even though our lives look quite different, she could hear herself in my story, and rather than it feeling like a self-indulgent exercise about me, it worked to support her growth. And for me, it boosted my self-esteem, too. Going back over the events of my adult life was good for me, because I started to see threads I'd not noticed before, I recognized that I had shown courage in moments when I could have stepped back, and it reminded me that things tend to work out eventually, even when it looks pretty awful at the time. "This is a podcast episode," said the client. I took her advice and recorded a section of my story on the podcast a few weeks later.[5]

Your story deeply matters. Not simply because it's your story (but that is reason enough), but because of the impact it can have on your growth and on the people around you. We've worked hard on your unique talents so far in this book, but they don't exist in a vacuum. They've been developed, refined, and tested throughout every season and moment of your life. Where our true strengths might be our fingerprint, our personal story reflects our heartbeat: constant and uniquely our own.

But why is this important? Reflecting on our story allows us to understand how past experiences, challenges, and successes have shaped our present selves. It helps us see patterns, recognize where we've grown, and pinpoint areas where we can continue to evolve. Without acknowledging our own narrative, it's hard to grasp the full picture of who we are and what we can become. It can give us the confidence to see ourselves in a new light, realizing we've been perfectly cast in the leading role from the start. And this understanding is crucial in the pursuit of purpose – because purpose isn't something that simply appears out of nowhere. It's the culmination of everything that has come before, a thread woven through your experiences, values, and the lessons learnt along the way.

By looking back at your story, you can start to see how it informs your future and how each chapter brings you closer to your true purpose. Every time I've shared my story, it has never failed to increase connection, confidence, and clarity – both for myself and others.

Coaching Notes: Bianca's Story

Bianca came to me for some coaching because, although she had climbed the ranks in her organization quickly and was well respected by her peers, she was keen to tune in more fully to who she was and what she did best. She sometimes found herself unsure, wondering if she was leading well, parenting well, and working well with others. There was, at times, a little voice undermining her capabilities, and she was keen to silence it. She knew she could do her job – that wasn't the issue. It was more that she wasn't sure what it was that she particularly contributed.

As we looked at her life story, we saw how events had shaped her. She talked about the highs and the lows, the big events and the memorable moments. Bianca had had an unusual childhood because of the nature of her father's career, which meant they had to live with a high level of security, and trust in the people surrounding them was non-negotiable. This explained Bianca's need for loyalty, honesty, and integrity, and why she placed trustworthiness above all other traits.

She'd also lived all over the world due to her previous work as a flight attendant, which had included some high-risk situations. Bianca's adaptability and capacity for risk had clearly been shaped by these situations. She was also quick to understand others, a skill she began to realize had been developed by all the speedy connections she'd had to make in this season of her life. Being a mother of three very different children with diverse needs had also given her many opportunities to grow the gift of awareness, too.

As we walked through the moments of Bianca's life, she could see the imprint they had left on her. The re-telling of her story made her stop and pay attention to it, as she could see how fascinating it was to me and how I could see themes emerging. "It's so easy to downplay your own story, thinking everyone else's has something more to it," she said. "I'm more aware than ever before how my life's experiences have developed me, shaped me, and pushed me." Bianca has a brilliant story, and now she could see it.

Activity: Your Timeline

How has your story formed you? It's time for your journal. Versions of this reflective activity are regularly used at the start of therapeutic work. I've done this myself and found it so helpful in spotting patterns, getting to know myself, and seeing how life events impacted me.

Step 1: Map your timeline

On a landscape piece of paper, I'd like you to simply draw a horizontal line along the middle, with the beginning of the line representing the beginning of your life (date it, if you like) and the end of the line being life right now (also date it, if you like). You will then think about and map out the events of your life, chronologically. These don't just need to be the huge ones like getting married and having a baby, although these should feature. It's up to you to put in as much detail as you like, anything that comes to mind or feels significant to you.

Step 2: Consider positive and negative events

Things that you felt were positive events, you will track above the line, and things that were negative you will track below the line. The further above the line you write the event, the more positive it was, and the further below the line, the more difficult the event. Some events are fairly neutral, so write those near the line. If it helps, you could brainstorm a list before committing it to your timeline.

Step 3: Take your time

You might want to come back to this and complete it in more than one sitting. When I did this activity, there were some obvious inclusions such as the big career changes I made, my marriage, and the birth of my children. Some other major life events were on the list – some neutral, some positive, and some that had been so hard at the time. Then there were other interesting memories that came to mind that surprised me, and had a bigger impact on me than I may have realized at the time. As I stood back from my own timeline, I could see how those events had shaped me and propelled my life in a certain direction; how they had not only grown my ability to connect and communicate but also contributed to some of my people-pleasing behaviours, too. More than anything, I could see how my story had helped make me who I uniquely am today (warts and all). I guess they formed part of my *poíēma*. I too am learning not to minimize my experiences but to make them part of my story and see how they add to my distinct contribution.

Step 4: Reflect

Once you feel like you're finished, here are some reflective questions to help you apply what you've done to our work on finding purpose.

- Can you see how your unique strengths from the previous activity were developed by some of these life events? Which ones?
- What do you feel your timeline says about the unique value you bring to the world? How can you embrace that more fully?
- If your timeline were the foundation for a new chapter in your story, what themes or lessons would you like to carry forward?
- Are there some aspects of your story that you have undervalued or undermined? Where have you shown courage or strength?

Note: It's important to stress that we are looking for themes and patterns to help us explore our unique contribution. I am not suggesting that it is okay that awful things happened to you, even if they have shaped you. If any of the things that you reflect on feel deeply painful and unresolved, please take this as a cue to consider reaching out and talking to a counsellor or therapist.

The Science and Soul of Storytelling

Once we have taken the time to recognize our unique story and acknowledge that we are perfectly cast in our own lives, we can begin to understand how important the stories we tell ourselves – and those we share with others – can be. Storytelling is powerful. At the time of writing, I've just watched the most brilliant ad for a car.[6] It starts with a couple finding out they are expecting a baby. Later, the woman leaves the house on foot, and the film cuts to the man chatting to his mum, sharing the wonderful news. He starts talking to her, imagining the future, which you can see developing in the footage being shown: this baby begins to grow, the little girl becomes a teen, then a young woman. The future dad is narrating the future he is imagining for himself, his wife, and his child, envisioning his hopes and fears. Every so often it cuts to the present day, with the newly pregnant woman walking along the road, approaching a pedestrian crossing. You can also see a car coming from a different direction, heading for the same crossing. The driver doesn't see the woman until the last moment. She puts her foot on the brakes, and the safety of the car means the accident doesn't happen. The future story that the man has been narrating has not been thwarted, it is safe to take place. It's incredibly moving. Subliminally you're taking in messages about why this is the safest family car, the car you need. But more obviously, you're drawn into a story we can all imagine. One of family and connection. Powerful stuff.

But what's going on? Why, in three-and-a-half minutes, have I felt such a range of emotions and a deeper connection to this car manufacturer? Well, it's the science of storytelling.

In his brilliant TED Talk, storytelling legend David JP Phillips explains that there is an "angel's cocktail" of good hormones – neurotransmitters – that are activated and released when we tell or hear stories, triggering positive emotions and quick physical responses in our bodies.[7]

It's quite amazing. First we have dopamine. The release of dopamine has a positive effect on the brain when we listen to a story. When it's in the blood, we are more focused, more motivated, and our memory is sharpened. When we hear the arc of a story and are waiting to hear what happens next, dopamine floods our body. Next, there's oxytocin. When this is released, we become more connected, more generous, and our trust is increased. This constitutes our emotional investment. When we hear and tell stories of our shared humanity and reality, oxytocin gets moving and this creates a deeper bond between us, and arguably with ourselves. David says that oxytocin allows us to feel empathy, to feel more human, and is therefore "the most beautiful hormone of all". Finally, stories release endorphins. Endorphins are known as "feel-good" chemicals because they can help relieve pain, reduce stress, and improve mood. When we hear happy endings, or about the wonderful moments of life, endorphins flood our system and not only do we feel happier, but we are also more creative, relaxed, and focused.

So, the proof is in. Crafting, writing, shaping, sharing, and listening to stories – our own and others – is good for us. It's how we get motivated, focused, connected, and creative. How we become more purposeful. Storytelling not only enhances our emotional wellbeing but also helps us clarify our values, goals, and aspirations. When we reflect on our own stories or share them with others, we begin to align our actions with our deeper purpose, making each moment more meaningful and intentional. This alignment happens because storytelling invites us to see patterns in our lives – the challenges we've overcome, the choices we've made, and the values we've upheld – helping us make more conscious decisions that reflect who we truly are.

Become the Hero of Your Own Story

Once upon a time, I was a primary school teacher. Learning to craft a good story is a large part of primary school writing, and so teaching children how to do that was a big part of my job. We used to use something called "The Hero's Journey" to help children grasp the key components they needed to include in their literary masterpieces. In his 1949 book, *The Hero with a Thousand Faces*, Joseph Campbell argues that every good story follows the monomyth, a set of events that must take place for the story to fully develop and then resolve.[8] Neither primary school children nor you and I need the full details, but an abridged outline is helpful. Here, I'm adapting from the classic mythological or mystical adventure story, so it fits with our everyday lives.

- First, there is always a hero. The main character, if you like. The main character begins the story in the "ordinary world" – life as they know it. They sense a call to a new adventure. For you and me, this could be the feeling that a new season is coming. But the hero resists the call. They want to stay with what they know, to stick with safety. Often at this point, someone (or something) comes along to help and act as a guide or mentor. Because of this intervention, our main character crosses the threshold and decides to step into the unknown.
- There follow tests, trials, and sometimes enemies who get in the way of our hero's progress, but with support they continue towards their goal. Sometimes the hero makes a mistake along the way – they act out of emotions such as fear, jealousy, anxiety, or insecurity. They take detours or find themselves stuck.
- Then comes what is known as the "ordeal". A significant challenge comes along that forces the hero to look at things differently, move on from the past, and step into their next season, a new version of themselves – they have grown. As they grow, they are rewarded with successes and opportunities, and they begin to make their way back – not to how things were, but onto the next phase of their journey, starting from a higher plateau.
- On the way back, when all seems well, that's when the final showdown takes place (we are often led to think that this has already happened). This is when the hero is once again confronted by their enemy (in our case this is likely to be self-limiting beliefs or roadblocks than an evil mythical creature). In this showdown, the main character defeats the "enemy" once and for all and is never the same again. They have changed for the better, and it is now time to celebrate, regroup, and enjoy the victory.

As I wrote this section, I found myself reflecting on my own journey so far. If I put myself in the story as the hero, I can see how my life has gone through a series of "quests" in the form of life events, decisions, and challenges. I can also see how situations and even people may have potentially thwarted my progress – and even succeeded in doing so – and how I have had to dig deep, with the help of trusted others, to get through to the other side. Recognizing these elements has helped me gain a deeper understanding of my own story and see how I've navigated setbacks and achieved growth, and where I might still need to step up.

This awareness allows me to make more intentional choices about how I move forward, ensuring that I embrace the next season of my life with more confidence and clarity. By applying the framework of the Hero's Journey to my own experiences, I'm able to better navigate the challenges ahead, knowing that each phase is part of a greater purpose-driven process. Soon, you'll have the opportunity to craft your own Hero's Journey, which will help you better understand the key moments and turning points in your life. But before you dive into that, let's explore some foundational storytelling principles that will give you the tools to tell your story with clarity and impact.

Make It Matter: How to Share Your Story

I love listening to a good story. A great story has an impact, whether it's over dinner with a friend and they're re-telling their latest faux-pas, or I've got my headphones in listening to a podcast or a book. I also enjoy telling a good story. I do it with my clients, in my work as a speaker, with my friends as we walk our dogs, and I even do it with strangers I meet.

I want you to be able to tell *your* story. I don't mean for you to sit down and download the entirety of your timeline to another person. I mean segments of your story – either seasons of your life or moments of your day. I want you to be able to do that with your family, your friends, at an interview (this is very important), as you lead others, and as you share your ideas. I admit that we aren't all natural storytellers, and that's okay. But only you can tell your story, and so having some key principles to work with will help you learn to do it in a way that connects, sparks people's minds, and inspires action. Here are some storytelling principles that will aid your prep and boost your impact.

Remember who you are talking to

When telling a story, it can be easy to forget the audience. It's so important to remind ourselves of who it is we are communicating with so that points of connection can be made. The same story can have different aspects highlighted so that it lands with whoever you're talking to. What should you emphasize? What should you leave out?

You need a core message

Whether we are telling a story to illustrate a point in an interview, or to explain a moral to a teenager, we need to know the core message. This helps us to ground what we are saying and not to go off on tangents, but also ensures we land the story on this point. What's the key point of your story? Can you distil it down to one line? Is there a moral you're trying to convey?

Start strong

The start of any story needs to hook someone in. We want to hold the listener's attention and get them to be quickly invested in the story we are about to tell. How can you start your story in a way that draws the listener in from the get-go?

Follow the arc

We've already talked about the Hero's Journey principles of a good story. Of course, there won't be all those elements in a story about a missed train, but it does need to have a clear narrative arc. Think of it more simply as including the following elements: an introduction or hook, the build-up, the dramatic moment, the tension falling, and then a conclusion. Can you plot your story along these lines?

Connect

The best stories involve emotional connection. Just think about the memes you bother to share. The best ones make us laugh, remind us of ourselves, get us to reflect, and bring tears to our eyes or a smile to our face. What's the emotion you're looking to evoke? How can you do this? When appropriate, a measure of vulnerability closes the gap between the teller and the listener. What does it feel like to be 10 per cent more vulnerable than you might otherwise choose to be?

Use your personality

Great storytellers come in different packages. There's absolutely no point in you trying to be me or anyone else; it never works and feels disingenuous. The best way for you to tell a story is to take on board the principles but do it in a way that reflects your personality. Think about the statements you came up with in the first activity of this chapter. How is that person coming across in your storytelling style?

Plan, practise, refine

Brilliant storytellers make it look easy. But even those of us who love to tell stories have to put the effort in. Collect stories and archive them for when they might be useful. Take the time to plan out a story so that the key points are heard, understood, and connected with. Look for cues from the listener so you can adapt or lean into different aspects next time.

✏Activity: Write Your "Hero" Story

For this final activity, I want you to take an event from your life that you would like to be able to share with others (and with yourself). Perhaps pick something that illustrates your personality or character, something that fits the hero story structure. Go through the six guiding principles above, ensuring you are the hero of this story, and then have a go at either writing the story out in full or recording a voice note of it if you prefer. Edit, improve, and practise, then share it with someone. It's also important to make sure you take time to reflect – what are the key threads in this story that weave together to help you see your unique purpose?

Key Takeaways

This chapter is called "The Waterfall" because, with its non-replicable formation and individual expression of nature, this acts as a metaphor for you. Your unique story and personality define you far more powerfully than external perceptions ever could. Recognizing your individuality helps you show up with confidence, connect authentically, and find your purpose. You are not "too much" or "not enough" – you are perfectly cast to play your part.

Your uniqueness stems from these truths:

- **You are irreplaceable:** like a Steinway piano, fingerprint, or waterfall, your combination of strengths, experiences, and attributes is one of a kind
- **Your story shapes you:** every event in your life – positive and challenging – has contributed to your growth and distinct perspective
- **Feedback is important, but not everything:** while the opinions of others can guide you, your true identity starts with your own understanding of yourself

To embrace your distinctive design, you need to:

- Get specific about exactly how to describe yourself
- Map out key life events to uncover the patterns and themes that shape who you are
- Let go of the fear of being "too much" and confidently step into every space as your authentic self

In short, your individuality is your strength. Embrace it, share your story, and see how it connects you to your purpose and the world around you.

Chapter Four

The Mountain

Recognize When You're at Your Best

Have you ever climbed a mountain?

When our boys were a lot younger, we decided we would attempt to climb Scafell Pike as a family. Scafell Pike is the highest peak in England, and for a young family it was quite the undertaking, especially for our youngest boy (he was five at the time), who was determined to keep up with his big brothers. Although my memories of the day are patchy, I know it was a lot of hard work, with plenty of motivational chat and chocolate along the way. There is one part of the day, however, that's etched in my mind, and that's reaching the summit. The sense of achievement, the relief, and the incredible sights. You've slogged and hiked and trudged for hours, but then you're rewarded with a breathtaking vista for miles around. You can see things that you couldn't see at ground level, and the new landscape shifts your perspective – it literally widens your horizons.

While you may not have climbed a literal mountain, I'm confident you've experienced some of your own peak moments. Let's take a metaphorical journey to that viewpoint now, reflecting on the highlight reel of your life so far. Alongside the absolute best bits, we'll also consider some of the admirable views you've encountered along the way – the everyday good stuff. Just like reaching the summit of a mountain gives you a new perspective on the landscape below, reflecting on both the extraordinary peak moments of your life, as well as the everyday good stuff, can offer valuable clues about what truly matters to you.

These moments, the ones that fill you with joy, fulfilment, or a deep sense of purpose, aren't random: they reveal patterns about what energizes you, what you're drawn to, and what makes you feel most alive. Sometimes it's the big, defining milestones, and other times it's the small but significant moments that quietly shape who you are. By paying attention to these highlights, we begin to see a bigger picture emerge, a landscape that helps guide us towards a deeper understanding of our passions, values, and ultimately our purpose.

Peak Moments

"Tell me about a time that you are really proud of."

This is something I always ask when beginning a new coaching relationship with a client. I'm looking for stories of the peak moments in their lives. A peak moment is a personal achievement that holds special significance for the individual, defined not by specific accolades but by its meaning to the person experiencing it. It's important that these moments aren't merely run of the mill, daily events, but are the highlights of our life so far, things that involved a significant measure of time, commitment, and enjoyment. When you stop and think about these moments, you know they challenged you, but in a good way that enabled you to use your strengths and grow in the process. Overall, you enjoyed them and gained satisfaction from them.

In summary, a peak moment memory can be any scenario, in any sphere of your life, that agrees with the following criteria:

- It stretched you
- You were at your best (using your strengths)
- It had meaning for you
- It energized you
- You enjoyed it

I'm reluctant to give a list of examples for this, because there are no right or wrong answers, and one person's example will be very different to another's. It's not just about the event itself, either – in fact, that's rather unimportant. What really matters is understanding the role that was played, the strengths and talents that were demonstrated, the feelings it evoked, and the difficulties that were overcome along the way. Reflecting on our peak moments is essential because it allows us to learn from them and intentionally shape our future. By celebrating these triumphs, we build a bank of memories that reveal patterns in our successes: what worked, why it worked, and what we did well. This reflection helps us define success on our own terms, rather than adopting someone else's version, enabling us to design a life and career that truly align with who we are.

One example of a peak moment in my own life was the first time I was asked to host a panel of experts at a women's conference. Let's look at why this fulfils the criteria of a "peak moment".

- **Stretching:** I'd done lots of live events before, usually giving talks or leading workshops, but this was the first time I'd been the host of a live panel, so it was definitely a challenge
- **At my best:** I got to use my talents in communication, quick thinking, and empathy throughout this event (and in the preparation beforehand)
- **Meaningful:** the topic was pursuing purpose, so you could say it had meaning for me!
- **Energizing:** in the moment I felt alive, not drained, and in my flow
- **Enjoyment:** afterwards, all I felt was "when can I do it again?"

Reflecting on peak moments allows us to uncover the true strengths, values, and passions that fuel us. By recognizing these patterns, we gain deeper insight into our unique purpose and can align our future goals and decisions with what truly energizes and fulfils us, creating a life of meaning and authenticity.

Coaching Notes: Rachel's Story

When Rachel began The Purpose Pursuit programme, she'd been in a season where she'd stayed at home with her young children. Before that, she'd worked in a school, for a charity, and for a start-up. This was all "BC" (before children), and her more recent years had been great in so many ways, but she wasn't sure she had any examples of "peak moments" to choose from. A lot of it had felt good, but more "everyday" in its nature, and I had banned her from choosing "gave birth" as one of the peak moments (yes, it's a major accomplishment, but I don't think it gives you much to work with for the purposes of this exercise). On top of this, she wasn't getting any inspiration from her previous work life, either. So, when she was working through this exercise, she drew a blank.

I encouraged her to think a bit wider, to be less binary about paid work and unpaid work, and to consider all the aspects of her life. For whatever reason, we seem to attribute less value to things that we don't get remunerated for, and yet they're often the things we hold most dear. "I did love it when we bought our home and renovated it," she realized.

As we talked, she could see how this had been a perfect opportunity for her to use her strengths. Was it a challenge? Absolutely – a tight budget and timeline and a lot of work to do. But Rachel is organized, creative, and great at connecting with people, and this project gave her the perfect opportunity to put those talents to work. She got the chance to project manage (she'd not done this in the workplace), show her creative flair, and work alongside a whole host of contractors that loved working with her and so always went over and above to make the project work. "It was a tough season at times, but it really was a time when I was in my flow. I guess I enjoyed the challenge because it pushed me to use these talents every day." The very definition of a peak moment. This knowledge boosted Rachel's confidence in her abilities and helped her think about what she needed in the next season of her life, recognizing she had a whole lot more experience in these fields than she'd first thought.

Activity: Your Peak Moments

Take out your journal and, using the guidelines I've suggested, stop and think about some of your peak moments from any season or aspect of your life – don't restrict it to work examples, unless you want to. For example, a non-work illustration of a highlight for me was when I performed as part of an orchestra at a national competition. Even though it was decades ago now, I can remember that day so clearly, and every time I hear an orchestra tune up it takes me back. This is an example of a peak moment for me because it gave me a chance to be pushed in the area of my strengths, as well as my love of performance, my natural enjoyment of music, and the emotion of the whole occasion. So make sure you think of work, play, education, and community. Any of these environments can have peak moments.

Once you've recounted some of the key elements of the event, here are some questions to ask yourself, reflect on, and coach yourself with. Don't feel you have to use them all, just pick those that resonate for you.

- **What strengths did I use?** Reflect on the specific abilities, skills, or qualities that you demonstrated during this moment. How did these contribute to the success of the experience? Think about the language you've been developing in the previous chapters.
- **How did I feel during and after the experience?** Reflect on your emotional state. Did you feel energized, proud, or fulfilled? What emotions come to mind, and what do they tell you about your passions?
- **What role did I play in this moment?** Consider the specific part you had in the event. Were you leading, supporting, creating, or innovating? How did this role align with your natural preferences and strengths?

- **How can I replicate this experience in the future?** Consider how you might intentionally create or seek out similar opportunities that align with your strengths, energize you, and provide meaning. Think about how this memory might influence your future goals, choices, or career trajectory. How can you build on this success?
- **What does this moment reveal about who I am at my best?** Reflect on the qualities, values, talents, and skills that shone through. How does this inform your understanding of yourself?

Scenic Stops: Everyday Highlights

As much as the moment on the mountaintop is important, the reality is that these instants are few and far between. We don't have peak moments every week; by their very nature they are standout occurrences – the absolute best bits – and don't happen in our everyday lives. The problem with only focusing on peak moments from the past is that although they do give us important feedback to work with, they don't tell the whole story. We need to examine our everyday experiences – the scenic stops on the way to the summit – because that's where we spend most of our time. Trudging up and down a mountain is a much bigger proportion of the trip than gazing at the glorious view from the top, so we need to make sure we're paying attention to what life looks like on an average day. On top of this, just focusing our attention on the peak moments can give us unrealistic expectations for our everyday life, and subsequently a whole load of disappointment to deal with, because our daily experience isn't matching up to the extraordinary moments from life so far. That's not to say that we can't improve our daily lives, for it is crucial that we work to do so – this is where we live out our days, so working to make them the best they can be is arguably more important than trying to chase the highs of the peak moments. In fact, the data backs this up.

Researchers and policy makers use something called "time-use data" to understand how individuals balance work, leisure, family responsibilities, and other aspects of daily life. Time-use data records the duration and sequence of activities people engage in throughout their day, along with contextual information like location, who they were with, and so on. They can use this data to spot trends and behaviours and then advise on policy or recommend reforms to help improve society. Now, if they go one step further and combine time-use data with subjective measures, they can see the impact of how we spend our time on our sense of wellbeing.

One such study tracked the use of everyday time, with correlating enjoyment scores to see how what we do in our daily life affects our sense of enjoyment, and in turn our wellbeing.[1] This study found that the higher the average for enjoyment of daily activity, the higher the overall life satisfaction score. So, the more we use our time in a way that we enjoy, the better we feel about our life and the better our sense of wellbeing. The ups and downs of regular life matter – it's not okay to have day after day with low enjoyment: settling for this means accepting a lower life satisfaction score and negative impact on our wellbeing. We need to tune in to our own "time-use data", tracking the parts of our day that we enjoy and the aspects of work that we prefer, and work to shift our time use so more of it fills the tank rather than takes from it.

Love What You Do?

There's a famous saying, "Find a job you love, and you'll never work a day in your life." Nobody is one hundred per cent sure who said it, but whoever it was, although I believe they meant well, inadvertently created a lot of pressure and potential for disappointment for most of the population. You might expect me to agree with this statement, based on the research we've just looked at. I do, in part, but I don't think it's phrased in the most helpful way and leads to misunderstanding as we seek to build a life that has purpose, meaning, and fulfilment. It creates the idea that those of us who have truly found work that we love won't *ever* feel like we are struggling, and that nearly all our time-use data will be full of high enjoyment scores. It suggests that life will be a utopian joy-fest, every day full of wins and energy, and we'll never have to do things that we don't like or find boring. It also makes people who don't love every aspect of their work (paid or unpaid) feel like they must be on the wrong path. It creates an unrealistic goal of finding unending love and excitement from every given moment, and if this somehow isn't the case, well, you've just not found your purpose yet.

I've got some good news for us all: research confirms that we don't have to be loving what we do *all* the time – just some of it. Better yet, this can be applied to paid or unpaid work. A study focusing on the wellbeing of nurses and doctors found a clue to life satisfaction and avoiding burnout in their time-use data.[2] They discovered that health professionals who spent 20 per cent of their daily time doing activities that they enjoyed seemed to protect themselves from burnout. If they crossed the threshold above 20 per cent, it seemed to protect them from burnout and move towards thriving at work. This 20 per cent needs to take place pretty much every day, as it doesn't work in the same way if we don't enjoy most of the week but like our Saturdays, for example. Each day needs to contain enough meaningful activities for us to experience greater life satisfaction and a positive sense of wellbeing. Let's identify what these things are, so we can increase the dose. Time to get out your journal.

Activity: Everyday Highlights

Step 1: Make a list

Using experiences from the past and/or events that are coming up soon, think about the things you have been doing that you have enjoyed. Get out your diary if you keep one or look at photos on your phone if it helps. We're looking to gather some time-use data, focusing solely on the enjoyable things we do in everyday life.

Remember that work, home, and leisure activities all count. It honestly doesn't matter how small the activity appears to be in your mind: if you enjoy it, write it down. Examples of the kind of thing we are looking for include: making lists, talking to new clients, going for a walk, tidying out a cupboard, doing the family finances, cooking a dinner, diary planning, decorating, reading, leading a meeting, brainstorming ideas, attending a team meeting, arranging flowers, telling a story.

Step 2: Ask why

Now that you have your list, ask yourself what you enjoy about these activities. Look beyond the surface to identify patterns and common themes. Which of your strengths and talents were being used? For example, if you like attending team meetings, what exactly about it do you enjoy? The ideas, the chat, or the action? Get specific and make a note of it.

Step 3: Reflect and apply

Don't skip this bit – there's little point in doing this activity if we don't look to see how we can apply the learning to our lives. Stop and coach yourself with these reflective questions. Don't feel you have to use them all, just pick those that resonate for you.

- What patterns or themes do I notice in the activities I enjoy? Are there common themes, such as working with people, being creative, or solving problems? Is it the process, the outcome, or the context (for example, working alone or in a team)?

- Which of my strengths or talents do these activities allow me to use? Consider what skills or natural abilities come into play when you engage in these activities. Do they tap into your problem-solving skills, creativity, leadership, or communication? Are you energized by analysing data, supporting others, or bringing ideas to life? How do they align with the strength types you identified in Chapter 2?
- How can I intentionally include more of these enjoyable activities in my daily schedule? Are there small adjustments I can make to my work, home, or leisure routines to incorporate more of what I love? What do I need to stop doing/reframe/delegate in order to do more of these enjoyable activities?
- How might I design my day to ensure at least 20 per cent of my time involves meaningful and enjoyable activities? What does a good day look like for me? What is one small change I could try today to test this approach? Is there someone I need to have a conversation with as part of my day shift? Note: if you're in paid work, at least 20 per cent of your work time should feel meaningful, not just the time outside of work. If you're a stay-at-home parent or doing unpaid work, aim for at least 20 per cent of your time to include activities you genuinely enjoy.
- What might my everyday highlights reveal about areas of my life I've undervalued? How can I make space to appreciate and nurture these moments more intentionally?

Trail Markers: The Gift of Feedback

So far, this chapter has focused on reflecting on when you think you have been at your best by considering your personal highlights; but when do others think you are at your best?

Earlier in the book, we briefly introduced the topic of feedback and why it matters, and how other people might spot our strengths before we do and be able to hold a mirror up for us, giving us clues about our true strengths and talents. Let's take that learning a little further now and zero in on what we uniquely do best.

Feedback is good for us. It's proven to help us to thrive, learn, grow, and feel valued.[3] Critical or directive feedback provides guidance, leading people to become, over time, more certain about their behaviour and more confident in their competence. But when our strengths and talents are highlighted to us, the impact is arguably even greater. A Gallup survey found that 67 per cent of employees whose managers focused on their strengths were fully engaged in their work, compared to only 31 per cent of employees whose managers focused on their weaknesses.[4] Positive feedback is one of the simplest ways to boost morale. I would go as far as to say the best feedback we can receive is when someone catches us being who we were made to be and tells us so – specifically.

Research shows that while nearly all of us agree that candid and insightful feedback is highly valued and necessary for our growth, many of us feel that the feedback we receive falls short of expectations.[5] We know we need it; we just don't always know how to receive it (or ask for it). It often ends up being woolly, non-specific, and hard to action. A generic "thank you so much" or "good job" means well, but, quite frankly, could do better. With some simple guidance, we can go on the hunt for meaningful feedback that can really shift the needle on our pursuit of purpose. It's time to be brave and get the kind of feedback that can make all the difference.

Coaching Notes: Anika's Story

Anika is a scientist who was enjoying her work in a broad sense, but her current situation regularly left her feeling frustrated and misunderstood. Her boss was good and fair, with no major issues, but just wasn't giving Anika the opportunity to use her true strengths on a daily basis. Here's a quick description of Anika: highly organized, detailed, fascinated by learning, responsible, loves to see people make progress, doesn't love conflict, and enjoys teamwork.

The problem was, Anika was having to work mainly on her own, in an unplanned and disrupted way, lacking ownership over how she worked. She really wanted to get involved in scheduling and planning but wasn't getting the opportunity to do this. She felt that her boss didn't understand her, and she wasn't sure how to shift the situation because of her preference for harmony over tricky conversations. She was wondering whether the only way through this was to just look for a new role.

We started working together, and instead of encouraging her to go straight to the job ads, I pushed her to do two things: to share her list of true strengths with her boss, asking for thoughts on them; and to ask her for some specific feedback on a highlight of her work so far. She was nervous to do this, but used our coaching as an excuse, sending over a request for feedback on her strengths and talents, and on a work project she had been involved in that had been a real positive for Anika, with great outcomes for the organization too. This is the message I got back from her:

"When I first spoke to her about it, I felt she was totally disinterested. But I followed it up with an email, and to my surprise I got a response back with a list of specific ways she could see my strengths and talents and how I particularly made that project a success. She commented on my project management, my desire to learn, my high levels of responsibility, and my ability to use time well. And here's the amazing bit – she now wants to talk to me about an upcoming project that she wants me to lead on because it would really fit with my strengths and interests. I can't believe how this exercise has prompted her to think differently about me. I also feel so much more affirmed in my work, and I feel more understood by my boss than I ever have before."

✏Activity: Why Me? Feedback

Pick a situation where you felt you were at your best. This could be a work project, a presentation, a home project, or something you were involved in as a volunteer. What matters is that you did it with someone else. Then, whether by email, text, phone call, or carrier pigeon (you choose), contact that person or persons and ask them to please help you with a self-development exercise. You will know how best to put it, but here are a few pointers to make sure the quality of the feedback is good:

Step 1: Frame the ask

Rather than just asking for a paragraph on who you are and what you do well, frame the request for feedback within a situation or scenario, the more recent the better. Examples could be, "Thinking about the time we worked together on the launch event", or "Referring specifically to the time we renovated the house".

Step 2: Give prompts

Most of us respond better to clear prompts, giving better quality feedback by breaking it down into responses to specific questions. Here's a few prompts you could use:

- What would you say was my core contribution?
- What is one thing I did especially well?
- How did my actions make a difference?
- Was there a specific moment where I stood out?
- How do you think my involvement influenced the outcome?
- What do you see as my greatest strength?
- How would you describe my unique contribution to a team or project?
- If you had to sum up what I bring to a situation in one sentence, what would it be?

Step 3: Ask them to keep it positive

This exercise is not designed for the collection of criticism or constructive notes on how you could have done better – there is a time and place for that, and this isn't it. I want these reflections to be positive only because, for most of us, if we hear the positive intermingled with the negative, we only remember the negative. Gently ask them to keep their responses focused on the what-went-wells, this time.

Having done this activity with lots of people, I know it can elicit a whole range of emotions. You could feel fear that you won't get a response, or that what they have to say doesn't sound like you. You could feel anxious that people will get the wrong impression of you, or maybe excited to hear what someone might have to say to you. All I can say is, go for it. Remember Anika – this exercise reaped so much more of a reward than she could have ever imagined. You might not get a response, and you might not like what they say. But you just might, too.

Key Takeaways

Your best self is revealed in both your peak moments and everyday highlights. These moments offer rich data about your strengths, values, and what energizes you. Peak moments are significant achievements that stretched you, showcased your true strengths, and brought you meaning and enjoyment. Everyday highlights, on the other hand, are the smaller, consistent activities that boost your daily wellbeing and satisfaction. This is the stuff we need to do more of to pursue our purpose.

True fulfilment comes from recognizing and intentionally integrating these insights into your life:

- **Peak moments:** reflect on standout achievements that challenged and energized you; identify the strengths you used and how they contributed to success
- **Everyday highlights:** track the daily activities that bring you joy, and ensure at least 20 per cent of your time is spent on meaningful tasks to protect you against burnout
- **Feedback matters:** seek specific, strengths-focused feedback from others to uncover patterns and affirm your unique contributions; be brave and discover the difference you make to others

When you understand and apply these insights, you can intentionally design a life and career that aligns with your true strengths, increasing your happiness, productivity, and overall sense of purpose.

Chapter Five

The Valley

Understand Your Weaknesses

You are your own worst enemy.

Annoying, isn't it? It's a tired cliché that we've all heard before, but could there be some truth to it? I'm afraid so.

Many of us are far too comfortable focusing on our weaknesses, flaws, and all the ways we could be better. Self-criticism comes naturally, and society only reinforces it. On top of that, it seems we are predisposed to remember the negatives over the positives, a phenomenon known as the negativity bias.[1] From performance reviews to personal development, the message is often the same: do better, and be better. That's why I've intentionally made you look closely at your strengths, your talents, and your standout moments first. Because before we talk about what you don't do well, you need the right foundation: a clear understanding of your own brilliance. (And yes, I hope you're getting more comfortable with that word – brilliant. Because it applies to you.)

But the reality is, we don't always get it right. We say things, do things, and make choices that don't help – sometimes for ourselves, sometimes for others. We frustrate ourselves by repeating patterns we wish we could break; seemingly self-sabotaging our own progress. And then there are the moments when our actions are misunderstood, misinterpreted, or misperceived – or is that just me?

But what's interesting is that we tend to look at weaknesses in the wrong way, and the very definition of a weakness leads us towards this conclusion. According to the Oxford English Dictionary, a weakness is "the quality or condition of being weak, in any sense of the adjective; deficiency of strength, power, or force."[2] In other words, it's something you lack. Something you need to fix because you're *bad* at it.

But what if our strengths – our talents and areas of real brilliance – could also be our weaknesses? In my experience, almost every challenge we face can be traced back to our strengths. William Shakespeare was onto something when he allegedly said, "Your greatest strength begets your greatest weakness." Honestly, the qualities that define who we are – the things we are hardwired to do – can be the real source of the challenges in our lives. The good news? This awareness is the starting point for change. Once we understand what's getting in our way and why, we can stop beating ourselves up over it and start using that insight to make real progress.

In Chapter 2 we explored key principles for identifying our true strengths. But there's another important factor to consider. A strength or talent is only truly a strength if it leads to positive outcomes – both for you and for those around you. A strength that isn't serving you well, or is negatively impacting others, in my book, isn't really a strength yet. For a strength to be truly effective, it needs to work in a way that is good for you and good for the people around you. If it's not doing both, then it's not a strength – it's just potential waiting to be refined. Let's look at these two areas in more detail: what makes a strength good for you, and what makes it good for others.

Part One: It's Got to Be Good for You

I'm thinking back to my teaching days. There was a time when I could hand-on-heart tell you that the very strengths of my personality were exhausting me. I held a leadership position in a school that was facing significant social deprivation. The school had been through a tough period and our team was on a mission to turn things around – to create an environment where children received excellent teaching and the best possible opportunities. I believed deeply in this vision, and my strong sense of purpose had found the perfect outlet (one of my top three strength types is the Believer).

When something matters to me, I give it everything: long hours, relentless effort, full commitment – no question. If that sounds self-congratulatory, I don't mean it to be. It's just something I've learnt about myself over the years: if I believe in something, I will pour myself into it completely.

But here's the problem. The way the world of work is set up, if you're willing to give your all, someone's willing to take it. Structures aren't designed to encourage balance and boundaries; they're designed to maximize output. And if the people around you are equally committed to the cause, they'll gladly take whatever you're offering – no questions asked.

That meant long days and even longer nights. My boys were young at the time, and I made sure to be home for teatime and bedtime. But once they were asleep, I'd open my laptop and start all over again. Pretty much every weekday night and every Sunday evening, the same pattern would repeat. Planning, marking, emails, and trying to do some of the bigger projects assigned to me. And I didn't do this begrudgingly: it mattered to me, and I genuinely believed I was making a difference.

But life happens. Things outside of work – big and small – started demanding more of my time and attention. And when you're already running at maximum capacity, even a small shift can tip the balance too far – sometimes it sent me crashing headlong over the edge. Add in the sheer exhaustion that comes from working at this pace, not as an exception, but as the norm, and it's a clear path to burnout – a burnout fuelled not just by circumstances, but by my very strengths and personality.

There's more to this story. Not only am I purpose-driven in my work ethic, but I am also someone who genuinely loves people. I honestly like pretty much everyone I meet, and I work hard to make friends with the people I encounter. My leadership style is open, warm, and friendly. You don't earn my trust: I freely give it until proven otherwise. I put a huge amount of energy into the relationships around me, not only because I like people but also (and here's the really honest bit) because I want them to like me. And herein lay the problem. I wanted my boss to like me, notice my efforts, praise me, and appreciate me. I wanted my team to like me, affirm me, and value me. What people thought of me really mattered.

And that's where things started to unravel.

This strength, my ability to connect with people, had gone into overdrive. It was leading my decisions, shaping my leadership, and taking up all my time. I found myself doing work that wasn't mine to do, answering emails at ridiculous hours, saying yes to extra responsibilities not just because I'm naturally enthusiastic, but because I wanted to be seen as helpful, capable, and indispensable.

Slowly, my decisions, my time, and ultimately my life became ruled by an overriding narrative around being accepted, appreciated, and liked. You could say that the volume on this aspect of my personality was turned up so loud it was doing me harm.

It was pretty deafening to be honest.

And when I finally hit burnout, I could see that it wasn't just the circumstances that got me there: *it was me*. And I wonder, as you read my story, if you're having your own similar realization. When we push our strengths too far, particularly when they become motivated by external validation, a need to prove ourselves, or the inability to stop, they can start to work against us, tipping the balance from productivity to exhaustion – and ultimately to burnout.

Burnout: The Slow Fade of Purpose

The unrelenting demands of work, the expectations of leaders, and the pressures of personal life create the perfect storm, making it harder than ever to stay healthy and flourishing. Nobody sets out to burn out, yet it's becoming a global epidemic, and the data is overwhelming. According to a 2019 Gallup study, 28 per cent of full-time employees reported feeling burnt out at work "very often" or "always". An additional 48 per cent reported feeling burnt out "sometimes".[3]

That means most full-time employees – nearly eight in 10 – at least sometimes experience burnout on the job. And it's showing no signs of going anywhere, in fact the data trends suggest it's on the up. Take British doctors as an example. Findings from the General Medical Council's 2022 national training survey revealed that 39 per cent of junior doctors reported experiencing burnout to a high or very high degree because of their work, and this is up six percentage points from the previous year's survey.[4]

But what exactly is burnout? Is it just feeling tired and needing a holiday? Is it the result of a stressful few weeks at work? No, it's much more than that. To truly understand burnout, we need to distinguish it from ordinary stress and exhaustion. Recognizing the difference is crucial, because only then can we see when we're at risk of falling into it.

Herbert Freudenberger first coined the term burnout in the 1970s, drawing from his own experiences as a clinical psychologist working with patients struggling with substance abuse. He noticed that he and his colleagues, despite their deep commitment and belief in their work, were becoming increasingly detached, disillusioned, and emotionally drained. The key point here? They believed in what they were doing, yet they were losing their motivation, energy, and drive. Their get up and go had got up and gone. Sound familiar?

In 1974, Freudenberger published his findings in a journal, marking the first time this phenomenon was formally recognized as burnout. He defined it as: "The extinction of motivation or incentive, especially where one's devotion to a cause or relationship fails to produce the desired results."[5]

Let's break that down into something more practical. Burnout has three key components:

- Emotional exhaustion: you're fatigued to your bone
- Depersonalization: you just can't bring yourself to care like you did – you're numb
- Decreased sense of accomplishment: your efforts seem futile, and nothing makes a difference

I wonder if you've felt this. Maybe you're feeling it right now. As you're reading this book, hearing my story, perhaps it's hitting a little too close to home. You can feel how exhausted you are. You know you're not functioning like you used to, and every attempt to get on top of your responsibilities just falls flat. Worse still, you're starting to realize that some of this exhaustion isn't just about what you do – it's coming from *who you are*. Your personality, your strengths – the very things that make you *you* – might also be what's running you into the ground.

If this is you, I'm so sorry. Life shouldn't feel this way. And I know that so much of what got you here isn't your fault and is outside of your control. Because the truth is, you can't just stop. You can't just leave work unfinished when there's more to do than there are hours in the day. You're not able to reply with an emphatic "no" when the list of patients outnumbers the hours left at work. You can't ignore emails from your boss, miss deadlines on important projects, or refuse to mark books (not without ramifications, anyway). It's not an option to stop feeding your children dinner or let the laundry pile up indefinitely. Your elderly parent still needs to be cared for, your teenager still needs a lift to and from their friend's, and your baby still has to have their nappy changed. For most of us, stepping back isn't an option. It's just not that simple.

And so we do the only thing we can: we keep going. We feel so out of control of the situation, we start to believe this is just how life is, and that there's no way out. We believe that this is adulthood; that we must suck it up and keep going.

But what if that wasn't the whole story? What if, instead of waiting for a major life overhaul (something I know some of you are seriously considering), you started with just a 10 per cent change? Would that feel more doable? Over time, a 10 per cent shift can transform your daily reality – creating more breathing room, more energy, and a renewed sense of purpose. And that shift starts with the one thing you *do* have control over: yourself.

Your personality, your motivations, and your mindset – the way you show up in the world – that's where real change begins.

Adjust the Volume

I want to suggest to you something that might be hard to hear. Sometimes, we're part of the problem. We may not realize it, but we are contributing to our own burnout. If you're feeling burnt out (or simply overworked and overwhelmed), chances are aspects of your personality have gone into overdrive. Think of your personality like a music mixing desk. Picture a row of channels, each with a sliding knob to adjust the volume. Each channel represents a different part of you, such as your drive, your empathy, and your attention to detail. The problem? If every knob is cranked up to full, the result isn't harmony, it's noise.

As you think about your own list, let's use mine as an example. My "channels" might be labelled like this:

- Belief-driven
- Enthusiastic kick-starter
- Quick-thinking problem-solver
- Wants to see people grow
- Enjoys meeting people and making friends
- Emotionally intuitive

Now, imagine that the sliding button on the channel is at max volume for each of these aspects of my personality, that I've cranked them right up to the top of the levels. How do they affect me negatively when I turn the volume up? Let me give you a clue:

- Belief-driven ⟶ Works myself into the ground
- Enthusiastic kick-starter ⟶ Takes on too many new things
- Quick-thinking problem-solver ⟶ Brain won't turn off, affects sleep and sense of peace and contentment

- Wants to see people grow → Ignores my own needs and growth
- Enjoys meeting people and making friends → Desperate to be liked and included
- Emotionally intuitive → Emotional exhaustion or heightened emotions that cloud my judgement

As you've read through this example, you may have started to reflect on your own "channels" and how they sound when the volume is turned up to the max. This is an important awareness to cultivate, and it will tie into our next reflection activity. You might want to grab your journal and note down your initial thoughts on this. Each of us has personality pitfalls that contribute to stress, exhaustion, and even burnout. Yours will be unique to you, but I hope that by sharing mine, I can encourage you (we're all in this together) and help spark ideas for your own list. But the important thing is – what can we do about it?

Recognize it

The first and most important step is simply recognition. Acknowledging our limitations – especially when they stem from our own personality, strengths, and talents – can be incredibly freeing. I'll go first:

"Hi, I'm Hannah. I have a habit of taking on too much, I can be overly emotional, and I have a propensity for people pleasing."

There, it's out in the open. I already feel better.

Make an action plan

Once we see the patterns, we can't just ignore them, we need a plan. But let me be clear: the goal isn't to erase these traits or become someone we're not. The goal is to refine who we are and to turn the volume *down*, not off.

Growth is not about a naturally empathetic person deciding they won't feel anymore, or an all-in, passionate person forcing themselves to be rigid and boundaried. Trying to shut down core parts of who we are can be just as damaging as burnout. This kind of behaviour can cause significant psychological distress and make us just as unwell as burnout, leading to dissatisfaction and disconnection. So don't try that. It is much healthier to be an increasingly whole version of who we are.

Let's use me as an example to show what an action plan looks like. I know my default mode:

- I say yes too easily, especially if I care about something
- I love starting new things and working hard for people I love (or like)
- My people-pleasing tendencies can push me to say yes when I should say no

So, here's my action plan to counterbalance these challenges:

1. I don't say yes (or no) immediately. I build in time – something I don't do naturally – to pause, reflect, and interrogate my intentions.
2. I ask myself key questions:
   - What exactly am I saying yes to?
   - Is this a good fit for me? Will it use my strengths?
   - If this commitment started tomorrow, would I still say yes?
   - What am I saying no to by saying yes to this? Because every yes is also a no to something else.
3. I seek perspective from trusted people. I have a few key people in my life who help me see what I might be avoiding. My husband Sam, my sister Keely, and my executive assistant Laura are great buffers for my overenthusiasm and over-commitment. They tell me the truth, even when I don't want to hear it. Who do you need in your corner?

Remember – this process isn't one-size-fits-all. This is *my* action plan, not yours. Maybe your challenge isn't saying yes too often, maybe you struggle to say yes at all. Maybe fear of failure or risk holds you back, leading you to say no to things that might actually help you grow. In that case, your action plan won't look like mine, it will involve pushing yourself to take *more* risks, not fewer. Reflect on your own action plan, working out what growth in this area looks like for you.

The key is self-awareness: knowing your patterns, understanding their impact, and making intentional choices that keep you thriving, not just surviving.

Coaching Notes: Holly's Story

When Holly came to me for coaching, she was recovering from severe burnout. Up until about a year before we met, she had been an exceptionally capable, highly experienced, and nationally award-winning palliative care nurse. She loved her job and knew she was good at it. She regularly went above and beyond – staying late, giving extra time, and ensuring the highest standard of care for her patients. She was so committed to this "over-and-above" mentality that she was given an award for it. Holly took immense pride in providing excellent care – not just for her patients, but also for their families, her team, and the wider system. She made sure every detail was right, every need was met, and every ball stayed in the air. Until one day, she simply couldn't do it anymore.

She described it as feeling like it came out of nowhere. There were no warning signs – at least, none she acknowledged at the time. On a particularly ordinary day, Holly went to work as usual, but at some point in her shift, she hit a wall.

"I can't do this anymore," she said to herself. And with that, she walked out of the building.

She never went back.

Holly hit burnout full force. She was signed off work, and eventually she handed in her notice, moving into a different area of nursing. It was at this point that she came to me, trying to figure out what had happened and what she should do next. She no longer felt the same way about work and was wondering if she needed to leave nursing altogether.

But let's take a step back. As you read Holly's story, I hope you saw what she later came to realize: her very strengths – the best parts of her personality – had gone into overdrive. She was wired for deep care, connection, and excellence, but when placed in a system that took everything she was willing to give, it led her straight to burnout. Her personality had contributed to her exhaustion, emotional depletion, and an overwhelming sense of futility.

Let's break down how Holly's very strengths became her weaknesses.

- *Natural emotional connection* ⟶ *Emotional exhaustion and depletion*
- *A problem-solving mentality* ⟶ *Self-critical, nothing is ever good enough*
- *Treating people as unique individuals* ⟶ *Disappointment with the generic system*
- *A deep sense of responsibility* ⟶ *Perfectionism, not saying no, over-committing, mustn't fail or let people down*

This knowledge was eye-opening for Holly. It helped her make peace with what had happened and, more importantly, show herself some compassion about why she had ended up there. But it also led to an unexpected realization. Holly had been searching for a way out of nursing, convinced that another career might suit her strengths better. And while there were undoubtedly other careers that she could easily undertake, she came to an altogether different conclusion: she was made to be a nurse.

Her strengths, talents, and natural instincts – when in balance – essentially defined what excellent nursing should look like. The challenge wasn't that she was in the wrong career. The challenge was learning how to bring her strengths back into balance, recognizing that while she couldn't change the system, she could change her response to it.

✎Activity: When Strengths Go into Overdrive

We've established that your strengths can also be your biggest source of stress and exhaustion, especially when they're running unchecked. The goal isn't to shut them down but to bring them into balance, ensuring they work *for* you, not *against* you.

This exercise will help you:

- Recognize how your strengths might be pushing you towards burnout
- Identify small but meaningful changes (10 per cent shifts) to regain control
- Develop an action plan that supports your wellbeing while staying true to who you are

Step 1: Identify your strengths in action

Using what you've learnt in previous chapters, list three to five of your core strengths. These could be from the strength types, personal reflection, or feedback you've received.

Step 2: Recognize when strengths go too far

Now, imagine what those same strengths look like when they're in overdrive. Your top strength types may give you some insight, so use the table on the next page to help guide your thinking (this is not an exhaustive list). Like previously, focus on your top three strength types.

Strength type	When it works for you	When it goes into overdrive
The Achiever: gets things done, thrives on results, enjoys ticking things off a list	Productive, goal-oriented, high standards	Workaholism, never switches off, feels guilty for resting, takes on too much
The Thinker: analyses, strategizes, seeks deeper understanding	Thoughtful, insightful, great problem-solver	Overthinks, struggles to make decisions, brain never switches off, mentally exhausted
The Connector: values relationships, creates a positive atmosphere, deeply empathetic	Supportive, great at building trust, relationally strong	Emotionally drained, prioritizes others at own expense, finds it hard to say no
The Impactor: inspires and leads others, confident in decision-making, takes initiative	Motivates, energizes, leads with vision	Pushes too hard, doesn't pause to recharge, feels pressure to always "be on"
The Believer: driven by values and purpose, committed to meaningful work	Passionate, dedicated, highly principled	Works to exhaustion, takes failure personally, struggles with compromise, self is low priority
The Explorer: curious, adaptable, loves new challenges and ideas	Open-minded, excited by possibilities, loves learning	Restless, struggles to commit, spreads themselves too thin

Take your own strengths list and write down what these look like in overdrive.

Step 3: Create a 10% shift

Pick one aspect of your personality that is currently exhausting you. Instead of aiming for drastic change, ask yourself, "What does 10% better look like?" This isn't about stopping being who you are – it's about tweaking the volume so it serves you better.

Here are some examples:

- **The Achiever** ⟶ Always working, struggles to rest
  10% shift: set a non-negotiable finish time and schedule one guilt-free break per day
- **The Thinker** ⟶ Brain won't switch off, always analysing
  10% shift: write down overthinking spirals and "close the loop" on your thoughts at the end of each day
- **The Connector** ⟶ Always putting others first, feels emotionally drained
  10% shift: set boundaries for emotional availability (for example, one "off-limits" evening per week)
- **The Impactor** ⟶ Always leading, feels pressure to be "on"
  10% shift: schedule personal time without obligations or expectations; schedule time away from meetings and availability
- **The Believer** ⟶ Feels responsible for everything, struggles with compromise
  10% shift: accept that not every problem is yours to fix: choose one thing to let go of
- **The Explorer** ⟶ Excited by new things, but spreads themselves too thin
  10% shift: set clear priorities and commit to finishing one thing before starting another

Step 4: Take action

Write down one small, doable action that you can take in the next week and month to make this shift happen. For example:

- My overdriven strength: The Achiever – I take on too much and never stop working
- 10% shift: set a firm stopping point each evening and practise guilt-free rest
- My first action: turn off notifications after 7pm and go for a walk instead

This isn't about fixing yourself, because you're not broken. It's about recognizing how your strengths impact your wellbeing and making small, intentional changes that help you thrive. Remember: a 10% shift today can lead to a radically different future.

Part Two: It's Got to Be Good for Others

When it comes to recognizing and working with the "dark side" of our personalities (yes, I know that sounds dramatic, but I do have a flair for that), there's another equally important aspect to consider: how we impact other people.

Your personality, in all its brilliance, is something other people experience, too. And I hate to be the one to tell you this, but it isn't always a wholly positive experience for them. The most obvious reason we might negatively impact others is when we simply behave badly. When our character (not personality – there's a difference) lets us down. When we act without integrity, maturity, kindness, or honesty. When we lash out, withhold, or let people down. You and I know what to do in these situations. We eat some humble pie, and we outright apologize and learn to do better and be better next time.

One of my non-negotiable beliefs is this: understanding your personality – your strengths, weaknesses, and quirks – is never an excuse for poor character. Good character trumps everything.

Personality is how you're wired, but character is a choice. And if you're reading this book, I'm guessing you already know that. But there are other, more subtle ways we negatively impact others, often without realizing it.

Under Pressure

What does your personality do when it is under pressure or stress? What happens to those wonderful strengths and talents of yours when the temperature of a situation is rising? I imagine, in the first instance, they serve you well. Organizers get busy bringing a plan. Doers start doing stuff. Innovators start coming up with solutions. Influencers start coordinating the response. This is all good. But what about a few more notches of stress and pressure? What happens then? Not always such a pretty picture. When we find ourselves in more pressurized moments (or days, or, let's face it, seasons) a distorted version of our personality can begin to emerge. We've already discussed how seasons of pressure and intensity can lead us to burnout, but what about how other people experience us when all is not fine and dandy?

I'm not so much talking about out-and-out awfulness. We've covered that. But just perhaps 10 or 20 per cent too much of a good thing? Ask yourself this: "When I'm at full volume, what does it feel like to be on the receiving end of me?"

Ouch. This question always makes me squirm a bit. Let's revisit our earlier examples.

Those organizers that get busy bringing a plan start moving towards rigidity, or my-way-or-the-highway behaviour. Those thinkers who bring creative solutions become blinkered to the impact of constant change on others, driving forward more and more changes that leave everyone else to play catch up; or the ideas keep coming and the implementation never happens. Those doers stop collaborating and work in powerful little bubbles, leaning into martyrdom. And the influencers tip into egomania.

Let's bring our examples a little closer to home. Under pressure, my natural instincts – quick decision-making, influencing others, deep empathy – start off as assets. But push me too far and suddenly my decisiveness turns dogmatic (I don't collaborate, I just decide), my influence turns controlling (I push too hard to get people on board), and my empathy turns over-emotional (I react instinctively instead of thoughtfully).

Now, what about if we come even closer to home? It's your turn.

- What happens to *your* personality under pressure?
- How does that impact the people around you?
- What small adjustments could help you find balance again?

These aren't easy questions to ask of ourselves, but if we don't start by asking, we definitely won't be able to make any changes.

At this point, you might be thinking, "Okay, I get it. I've done the self-awareness work before. I know my strengths, my weaknesses, and how I show up in the world." And to that, I'd say: Really? You've finished it?

I once worked with a senior leader who, just as we were about to start discussing personality challenges and blind spots, confidently told me, "Ah, thanks, but I don't need to do that stuff. I've done it already." Essentially, he was saying he had ticked the "self-awareness" box and didn't need to revisit it. If only it were that easy. But the truth is, the moment we think we've "completed" self-awareness, we've actually drifted the furthest from it.

This work isn't something you finish: it's a lifelong process of reflection, feedback, and growth. Yes, we make progress. Yes, we develop healthier patterns. But unless you're a perfect human being (and I'm willing to bet against that), there's always work to be done. Understanding your strengths and weaknesses through this ongoing process not only helps you grow but also allows you to make more intentional choices – aligning your actions with your values and ultimately leading a more purposeful life.

Misunderstandings and Misperceptions

"You're such a social butterfly, Hannah." I remember an old friend saying this to me, and she didn't mean it as a compliment. She saw my ability to quickly connect with people and make new friends easily as flaky, shallow, and attention-seeking. She assumed my enthusiasm was superficial – that I was just seeking external validation.

Ouch.

Was she right? Not exactly. But here's the hard truth: people's perceptions of us – whether we like them or not – are their reality. This doesn't mean every judgement someone makes about you is accurate, or that what was perceived was our intention or motivation. Far from it. But it does mean that how people experience us matters. It matters because purpose – the very point of this book – cannot be pursued in a vacuum. It thrives in connection, collaboration, and community. Understanding how others perceive us allows us to navigate relationships more intentionally, ensuring our actions align with the impact we hope to create in the world.

Second, perceptions are powerful: what other people are perceiving feels incredibly real to them. We humans form perceptions quickly and hold on to them tightly. There's a concept known as "thin slice judgements" that suggests that humans can derive meaningful information from very brief interactions – a quick glance, the way we smile, the kind of handshake that we give, a slight gesture – any of these actions gives us a lot of data in which to form a perspective.[6] So, when we behave in certain ways, or act in ways that are perhaps different to the person who is observing us, these thin slice judgements develop. That doesn't make them wholly accurate, of course. Cognitive bias, previous experiences, projection, personality differences, and all manner of defence mechanisms play into these opinions. The same goes for us, too – whenever we form a perspective on someone, it's not on a blank slate – our history, personality, life experience, and perhaps even stereotyping can be the base layer on which we build.

The point is this: sometimes people misunderstand us not because we've done something wrong, but because they're interpreting our personality differently from how we intended. It occurs all the time, and it's nowhere near as personal as it feels when it's happening. This is where understanding our weaknesses becomes so important. When we recognize the aspects of ourselves that might be misread or misunderstood, we give ourselves the chance to bridge the gap between how we intend to show up and how others perceive us. We can't entirely stop people from misunderstanding us – misinterpretation is a natural part of human interaction. But this isn't just about avoiding misunderstandings for their own sake; it's about ensuring that these moments don't create barriers to connection, collaboration, or community. After all, purpose – the very heart of this book – requires us to engage meaningfully with others. By addressing how we're perceived and working to align that with our intentions, we strengthen our ability to build relationships that support our goals and values.

So what *can* we do? By recognizing that misunderstandings will happen and taking proactive steps to address them, we can reduce their impact and create more room for meaningful connection. Here are some practical ways to approach this.

Pre-empt misunderstandings

Forewarned is forearmed, as they say. This book is designed to help you understand who you are – your strengths, talents, and preferences. But along the way, it also gives you the opportunity to uncover something just as important: how others might perceive you. By stepping into someone else's shoes and considering how they might interpret your behaviour, you can start to recognize the key ways in which you might be misunderstood. This isn't about changing who you are – it's about gaining awareness so you can navigate interactions with more clarity and intention.

Since we all love a good case study, let's use me as an example again. Taking the same strengths we explored earlier, let's now consider how they might be misinterpreted by others, whether they've just met me or have known me for years.

- Belief-driven → Self-righteous
- Enthusiastic kick-starter → Impulsive
- Quick-thinking problem-solver → Opinionated
- Wants to see people grow → Pushy
- Enjoys meeting people and making friends → Shallow
- Emotionally intuitive → Irrational

Identifying these patterns helps remove the sting when misperceptions happen – because you'll already know where they might come from.

Explain, don't excuse

There's a phrase I picked up not that long ago that I really like, and that fits well with this topic: it's an explanation, and not an excuse. It's very easy to fall into the trap of just excusing ourselves from doing better by declaring passive statements such as, "Well, I can't help it, it's just who I am." Or "Don't expect me to do such and such, it's just not in my nature." These kinds of opinions lack any sense of ownership or desire to do or be better. They suggest that the entire responsibility lies with the other person to just understand that this is who we are, and we won't give an inch. It's an excuse, without any personal accountability for the impact they may be having on other people.

Now, I'm not suggesting we simply roll over or take full responsibility for how others perceive us. Perception isn't always reality. Sometimes, despite our best intentions, people misunderstand us for reasons entirely outside our control. But there's a middle ground between outright denial ("That's not my problem") and total blame ("It's all my fault"). That middle ground? Explanation.

Once we recognize how we might be perceived, one of the most valuable skills we can develop is learning to communicate that clearly. By offering context and being open about our tendencies, we can help others understand us better – and even invite them to gently call us out when we might not see our own blind spots in the moment.

For example, I can talk the hind legs off a donkey; a fact that hasn't gone unnoticed. Some people might see this as a sign that I'm a poor listener, or – in the immortal words of my maths teacher, Mr Mills – that I have *verbal diarrhoea*.

What's *not* okay is shrugging it off with, "Yeah, I interrupt people – I can't help it. That's just me." Equally, I don't need to swing to the other extreme, drowning in guilt, vowing never to speak in meetings again (yes, I've been there too). Instead, I can offer an explanation, like this:

"I know I have a tendency to tell one story too many. I love a good chat, and my brain fires off ideas quickly, which sometimes means I accidentally speak over people. I don't want you to think I'm not interested in what you have to say, so if I'm going on too much, or I've been butting in, just give me a nudge."

This way, I own my possible shortcomings,.and without completely bending myself out of shape and not being who I am, I find a way to just be honest about it, explain it, and move on.

Each of these actions helps us navigate perceptions more intentionally, ensuring that our blind spots don't hold us back but instead become opportunities to deepen understanding and connection with others.

The Dark Side: More Than a Perception

Sometimes, the ways we irritate others – the habits that grate, frustrate, or wear people down – aren't just misperceptions. They're not simply the result of stress or pressure, either. And no, it's not because we've suddenly become terrible people. It's because of the dark side of our strengths. "There's an Achilles' heel to being you, Hannah," my therapist once told me.

There's an Achilles' heel to being you, too.

Even if you know the body part, you might not know the story. So let me indulge you. Achilles is a figure from Greek myths and legends. He was the alleged hero of the Trojan War (basically a battle between nations that started with a fight over the love of a beautiful woman). Legend has it that his mother, wanting to make him invincible, dipped him into the River Styx – a sacred river believed to grant protection. But there was a flaw in her plan: she held on to him by his heel, leaving that one spot vulnerable. And that's the part of the story that really sticks.

Achilles wasn't remembered for his strength, skill, or power. He was remembered because of his one weak spot: the heel that made him fall. When the Trojan prince Paris shot an arrow into it, Achilles was defeated. His strength wasn't enough to save him from his weakness.

And that's the lesson for us, too. Our strengths – our biggest assets – can also be our greatest liabilities when they tip too far. When that problem-solving skill becomes criticizing negativity. When the positivity turns toxic. When your desire to do things excellently becomes relentless perfectionism. When your self-assuredness leans into arrogance. In these moments we need to listen, take note, hear the feedback, and learn to steer ourselves away from the weakest aspects of our personality.

When this stuff happens, we just need to hear it, own it, and course correct. Here's a great question to ask yourself: what does it feel like to be on the receiving end of you? If you can answer that honestly, you're already on the path to growth and balance.

Coaching Notes: Tom's Story

Tom, a senior leader in his organization, came to me for coaching because of strained relationships with his team. Truthfully, he hadn't sought out coaching himself; it was suggested after growing concerns that, despite his positive impact, team tensions were beginning to outweigh the benefits of his leadership. Complaints and frustrations were surfacing, but Tom couldn't understand why.

As we worked together, Tom and I started with getting clear on who he was at his best. It became obvious to me that Tom prided himself on hard work, honesty, fairness, and going above and beyond. He set high standards for himself and others, believing that clear systems and policies provided structure and fairness for everyone. But that wasn't always how it was received. Some of the tension stemmed from personality differences between Tom and his team. Some of it was misperception. But some of it, quite frankly, was the dark side of his strengths.

The feedback told a different story. His high standards sometimes felt unattainable, leaving his team discouraged. His strong sense of fairness could come across as rigid and impersonal, overlooking individual circumstances and opinions. His dedication to doing things well led to a perception that he didn't trust others to do them right, so people stopped trying.

Tom was frustrated – his intentions were good, so why weren't they recognized as such?

To help him gain clarity, instead of focusing on specific situations we explored how his personality's Achilles heel might feel to someone wired differently. When he let go of defensiveness and took a more vulnerable approach, he began to see how his leadership – while built on strong values – was unintentionally creating frustration, hurt, and even resentment in his team.

Of course, this wasn't resolved overnight. Recognizing our own impact is hard. It's far easier to justify our actions than to change them. But this first step – acknowledging how his strengths were showing up at full volume – helped Tom create a plan. No one expected him to stop caring, lower his standards, or abandon structure. But what would it look like to use his strengths more intentionally – at the right time, in the right way, and in the right amounts?

Which brings us back to the mixing desk metaphor; when every channel is maxed out, all we get is noise. But with balance? That's when things truly start to work.

A final thought on how others see us. You might have reached the conclusion that it doesn't really matter what people think of you. After all, society, social media, and plenty of so-called gurus push the idea that you should "be who you want to be – it's nobody else's business". And like all bold statements, there's some truth in it. You *should* be who you are. If you're quiet and reflective, embrace it fully. If you're quick-thinking and love storytelling, share your ideas. If you're analytical and logical, let those strengths shape decisions. And if you're intuitive and emotion-driven, trust your instincts and share them.

But if this mindset leads us to believe that other people's perceptions don't matter at all, that's a step too far. We don't exist in isolation, and how others experience us *does* shape our relationships, our impact, and our development. It's how we grow. And by the way, it's a lifelong endeavour.

✏Activity: How Do Others Perceive You?

We've explored how our strengths, when in balance, are powerful forces for good. But when they're in overdrive – whether due to stress, pressure, or the way others perceive – they can become obstacles, not just for us but for those around us.

This exercise will help you:

- Recognize how your strengths might be perceived (or misperceived) by others
- Identify patterns that might be causing tension or misunderstandings
- Develop small but meaningful shifts to improve how you show up in relationships

Step 1: Identify your strengths in action

As in the previous activity, using what you've learnt in previous chapters, list 3–5 of your core strengths. These could be from the strength types, personal reflection, or feedback you've received.

Step 2: Consider how others experience your strengths

Now, reflect on how these strengths might be perceived or misinterpreted by others when they are running at full volume. Your top strength types may give you some insight, and so use the table below to help guide your thinking (this is not an exhaustive list!).

Strength type	When it works for you	How others might perceive it
The Achiever: gets things done, thrives on results	Productive, goal-oriented, high standards	Bossy, rigid, prioritizes tasks over people, impatient with slower processes, solo performer
The Thinker: analyses, strategizes, seeks deeper understanding	Thoughtful, insightful, great problem-solver	Overly critical, detached, overcomplicates things, slow to act, dismissive of emotions

Strength type	When it works for you	How others might perceive it
The Connector: values relationships, deeply empathetic	Supportive, builds trust, relationally strong	Over-involved, lacks boundaries, overly sensitive, plays favourites, emotionally intense
The Impactor: inspires and leads others, confident decision-maker	Motivates, energizes, leads with vision	Pushy, controlling, dominates conversations, doesn't listen enough, too intense
The Believer: guided by values, driven by purpose	Passionate, committed, highly principled	Self-righteous, unwilling to compromise, judgmental, hard to challenge
The Explorer: curious, adaptable, loves new challenges	Open-minded, excited by possibilities, loves learning	Unfocused, inconsistent, hard to rely on, jumps from idea to idea, avoids commitment, doesn't listen to risks

Write down how your strengths might be perceived by others, especially in times of stress or when they go unchecked.

Step 3: The reality check

Choose one strength that seems to cause the most tension or misunderstanding in your relationships. Reflect on the following:

- How might this strength be showing up in a way that frustrates others?
- Have you ever received feedback (directly or indirectly) that reflects this?
- Are there particular situations or people where this happens more frequently?

Step 4: Adjust the volume: create a 10% shift

Rather than overcorrecting and losing what makes you great, focus on small, intentional shifts – just a 10% adjustment – that helps your personality land better with others. Here are some examples:

- **The Achiever** ⟶ Can come across as rigid and task-focused
  10% shift: build in pauses to check in with people before pushing forward with tasks
- **The Thinker** ⟶ Can be seen as overly critical or slow to act
  10% shift: balance analysis with timely action; acknowledge others' ideas before refining them
- **The Connector** ⟶ Can feel too intense or emotionally involved
  10% shift: be mindful of emotional energy; ask before offering deep personal support
- **The Impactor** ⟶ Can feel pushy or overbearing
  10% shift: intentionally pause in conversations; invite input before driving decisions
- **The Believer** ⟶ Can come across as rigid or uncompromising
  10% shift: be curious about others' perspectives before jumping to conclusions
- **The Explorer** ⟶ Can be seen as inconsistent or distracted
  10% shift: follow through on one commitment before moving to the next big idea

Write your own 10% shift plan:

- The strength that sometimes creates tension: for example, the Achiever – I'm always busy getting things done
- How I think others might experience it: for example, my family might feel like I prioritize chores and tasks over spending quality time with them
- 10% shift: for example, intentionally pause and be present, even when there's still "stuff to do"

- My first action: for example, set aside 15 minutes after dinner to sit and chat without multitasking

Step 5: Invite feedback

One of the best ways to check whether you're improving is to ask the people around you how they experience you. Who do you trust to give you honest feedback?

Consider asking:

- When I'm at my most intense, how do I come across?
- What's one small thing I could do that would make working with me easier?
- Is there a way I sometimes misread or misunderstand how I'm being perceived?

Final thought: your true strengths are your greatest asset. But without fine-tuning, they can push others away or create tension. By recognizing when they go too far, and making small but intentional adjustments, you'll not only improve your relationships but also create a more sustainable way of showing up in the world. When your strengths are balanced and your relationships thrive, you remove unnecessary barriers and open the door to deeper connection, collaboration, and fulfilment – essential foundations for living a purposeful life.

Key Takeaways

Your greatest strengths are often the very things that create the biggest challenges – for you and for those around you. A strength is only truly a strength when it works in a way that benefits both you and the people around you. Otherwise, it's just potential waiting to be refined.

- Your personality can be a key factor in burnout, exhaustion, and frustration – especially if your strengths are running unchecked
- Other people may struggle with aspects of your personality for three key reasons:

- **Stress and pressure**: when we're overwhelmed, our strengths can tip into overdrive
- **Misperceptions and misunderstandings**: the way we see ourselves isn't always how others experience us
- **The "dark side" of strengths:** without self-awareness, our best traits can become our biggest liabilities

The best way to mitigate these challenges is through intentional self-reflection. Take responsibility, make a plan, learn to communicate your tendencies, and stop using your personality as an excuse for unhelpful behaviour. Less excuses, more explanation.

Your personality should be working for you, not against you. And when your strengths and talents have been fine-tuned, they become a force for real impact – both in your own life and in the lives of those around you.

Chapter Six

The Desert

Overcome Self-Sabotage

Do you ever find yourself behaving in ways that go against your best interests, even when you know better, when you don't even *want* to? Maybe you've stepped back from a job opportunity because you're not sure you're qualified enough, or maybe you've found yourself endlessly scrolling through a social media account that only leaves you feeling worse about yourself. Perhaps you've given up after the first attempt because you didn't nail it perfectly, or said yes to something that, deep down, you knew you should have declined. These are all examples of self-sabotaging behaviours, and they happen to the best of us. Just this past week, I've self-sabotaged in several ways. I procrastinated over writing parts of this book, putting myself under unnecessary time pressure. I compared myself to others and, predictably, found myself falling short. I even made choices I didn't want to make, purely out of a need to people-please. You make plans and set intentions to move towards the life you're looking for – and then, inexplicably, you pick up a wrecking ball and swing it straight at them.

Self-sabotaging behaviours drain us of energy, leaving us depleted, frustrated, and stuck, unable to move forward. It's like standing in the middle of a barren desert, where nothing can grow. And the hard truth is this: no one else is to blame – it's down to you. By swinging that wrecking ball, you keep yourself stranded in that dry, lifeless expanse where growth feels impossible. But before all hope is lost, here's the good news: there's an oasis in this desert. It comes in the form of recognizing these self-sabotaging behaviours, understanding why we engage in them, and creating actionable plans to think and act differently. With practice and intention, we can break free from these patterns and replace them with healthier habits – ones that allow us to build a life of purpose that's not only good for us but also benefits those around us.

In this chapter, we will focus on four common ways that we self-sabotage: feeling like an impostor, comparing ourselves to others, having a fixed mindset, and people-pleasing. For each, we'll unpack the problem, uncover the underlying issues, and work out why we do what we do. We'll then develop a personalized plan to shift not only the behaviour but the thinking behind it. My goal isn't to push you to become someone you're not. Instead, I want to help you grow healthily into the person you were always meant to be.

Self-Sabotaging Behaviour 1: Feeling Like an Impostor

Not long after leaving teaching and early in my new career as a coach and speaker, I was given my first big opportunity: speaking to a group of business owners about leading from a place of strength and talent. I was thrilled and threw myself into diligently preparing my workshop.

When the day arrived, I wore my best confidence-boosting outfit and caught the train into central London. The venue was something else – a swanky private members club for people who, at least to me, seemed worlds apart from who I was. I walked in, trundling my wheelie case behind me, and headed for the lifts. I remember the next moment vividly, even though it happened nearly a decade ago. As the lift doors closed behind me, I pressed the button for my floor and caught sight of my reflection in the mirrored walls. In an instant, six sharp words cut through my internal monologue:

"Who do you think you are?"

The words hit me hard. They had power and I believed them. In that moment, I felt the grip of impostor syndrome around me. I couldn't think straight, and my mind raced with all the reasons why I didn't belong there. I wasn't experienced enough, I didn't deserve this opportunity, I had nothing new or unique to offer this audience. My heart pounded in my chest, my palms grew clammy, and I had about 20 seconds before the doors would open to pull myself together.

This is impostor syndrome – or, as some call it, impostor phenomenon. I prefer the term "impostorism". A syndrome sounds incurable, and a phenomenon makes it sound like the Northern Lights, neither of which seem fitting to me. The concept is well known these days, but it was first coined by two clinical psychologists, Dr Pauline Clance and Dr Suzanne Imes, in the 1970s. Their original work focused on women, but it's important to make clear that although women seem to be more susceptible, it's not a women-only issue. Clance and Imes wanted to describe what they had discovered from interviews with 150 highly accomplished women who, despite earning advanced degrees, receiving academic honours, achieving significant milestones, and earning remarkable praise and professional recognition, felt no internal sense of success and saw themselves as impostors. Clance and Imes labelled this experience the "impostor phenomenon".[1]

According to Clance and Imes' seminal paper, impostorism is characterized by three key traits. First, there's the belief that others overestimate your abilities. Second, there's a fear of being exposed as being less capable than you appear. Finally, there's a persistent habit of attributing success to external factors, such as luck or excessive effort, rather than your own competence. This feeling often arises when taking on a new job or additional responsibilities, like in the story I shared from my own experiences. Ironically, the fear of being a fraud can drive people to work harder and be more conscientious, leading to greater success and advancement – which then fuels yet another cycle of impostor feelings.

It doesn't matter how accomplished you are, imposterism seemingly strikes without rhyme or reason. Sheryl Sandberg, Harvard graduate and former COO of Meta, confessed to her own sense of imposterism in her book, *Lean In*: "Every time I took a test, I was sure that it had gone badly. And every time I didn't embarrass myself – or even excelled – I believed that I had fooled everyone yet again. One day soon, the jig would be up."[2] Seth Godin, award-winning author and entrepreneur, admitted in his blog, "Yes, you're an impostor. So am I and so is everyone else."[3] While it might not quite include everyone, research consistently shows that most of us are affected. You and I, and most of the people we know – whether friends, family, or colleagues – are likely to experience moments of doubt, when we question whether we truly belong, deserve our position, or have what it takes. In other words, having these thoughts is normal. But that doesn't mean that they have the right to take up residency and sabotage our progress or sense of purpose.

Back to my story. When the lift doors opened, I made a beeline for the ladies' room. Standing in front of the mirror, I paused and gave myself a silent pep talk: "Hannah, in many ways you might feel out of place here. You don't speak the same way. You didn't grow up in this world, and your experiences are different from those of these leaders. You won't do a perfect job."

But then I reminded myself: "You have something no one else can offer. You bring experiences that are uniquely yours, a style that belongs only to you, and an approach that only you can deliver. Yes, there are others who *could* lead this workshop, but only you can bring your perspective, your voice, your authenticity. Lean into that. You can't be an impostor if you're being you."

Okay, in reality my pep talk was not that eloquent – but these are definitely the words that I needed to hear in that moment.

Impostorism and Your Personality

Impostorism doesn't look the same for everyone, it takes different forms depending on our personality, strengths, and insecurities. These variations, or "types", reflect our unique vulnerabilities and the ways we experience self-doubt. Identifying the type we relate to most helps us move beyond a one-size-fits-all approach, giving us clarity on what's driving these feelings: whether it's fear of failure, the need for validation, or unrealistic self-expectations. This self-awareness is the first step towards breaking free from the cycle of doubt and second-guessing. It also reveals how impostorism shapes our behaviour, from overworking and struggling to delegate to avoiding new challenges altogether.

External pressures can further intensify these feelings. Women, ethnic and religious minorities, and other underrepresented and marginalized groups often face added layers of expectation and biases, making the need to "prove" themselves even stronger. Recognizing these influences allows us to focus on what we can control while also pushing for broader change. Let's now take a closer look at how impostorism shows up in our lives so we can understand its impact and start creating meaningful ways to move past it.

Dr Valerie Young is a leading voice in the field of impostorism and was one of the first to recognize that it can manifest in different ways. In her work, she identified five distinct types of impostorism, or what she calls competence types, highlighting the diverse ways people experience and cope with feelings of inadequacy.[4] Building on her foundational work, I've developed my own approach to understanding impostorism. By narrowing it down to four types and using language that resonates with my personal experiences and observations, my aim is to make this concept even more accessible and relatable for you.

1. Must be perfect

You believe that every task you complete, whether it's at work or home, must be faultless. Your sense of self-worth is tied to the quality of your work or the standard you set. Any mistake, no matter how small, feels like a failure, which can lead to constant frustration or even avoidance. You often find yourself obsessing over the tiniest details to ensure everything is just right.

Work example: you're preparing a presentation for work. It's going well, but you keep reworking the slides, tweaking the wording, and adjusting the design because you're worried that if it's not perfect, your colleagues or boss might think less of you. You can't move forward because you're paralyzed by the thought of imperfection, even though you've already done the work and are ready to present.

Home example: you're hosting a dinner party and feel that everything must be flawless. The table setting needs to look like a Pinterest board, the food needs to be restaurant-level quality, and everything must go exactly as planned. When you realize you're running out of time or one dish doesn't look perfect, you start to panic, even though your guests won't notice the small flaws.

Not sure if this applies to you? Ask yourself:

- Do you struggle to move forward because you keep tweaking things, even when it's already good enough?
- Do you find yourself stressing over small details that others wouldn't even notice?

2. Must juggle it all

You feel like you need to excel at every role, whether it's at work, home, or in your personal life. You often take on too many responsibilities, thinking that if you can juggle it all, it proves your worth and purpose. You think people will be impressed by all the plates you have spinning in the air. However, this often leads to burnout and feeling overwhelmed as you try to juggle it all yourself. Hello, multi-tasking super person.

Work example: you're managing several projects, answering a stream of emails, and attending back-to-back meetings. As you try to finish a report, you're also trying to troubleshoot an urgent issue that popped up with a colleague, all while preparing for a big presentation later in the week. You're constantly switching between tasks and never really feeling like you're fully present in any of them. Even though you're exhausted, you keep pushing forward, thinking that if you just work harder and faster, you'll get everything done.

Home example: you're hosting a dinner party, but you're also trying to manage everything else. As you're cooking dinner, you're simultaneously trying to clean the living room, pick up the kids' toys, and answer a work email that came in. The laundry needs folding and your phone is buzzing with messages from friends about the party. You're bouncing between tasks, moving from one to the next without truly focusing on anything, all the while feeling the pressure to get it perfect. It feels like there's no end in sight, and you can't stop until everything is checked off your list.

Not sure if this applies to you? Ask yourself:

- Do you find yourself constantly multitasking, trying to juggle multiple responsibilities at once, even if it leaves you feeling drained?
- Do you get stressed when you're not working and find downtime completely wasteful?

3. Must know it all

You feel like you need to know everything before you take any action, whether it's at work or home. You tend to research, prepare, and learn endlessly, thinking that knowledge is the key to success. However, this need to know it all often holds you back from taking the necessary steps to move forward, because you rarely feel you know enough, even though you're already capable.

Work example: you're asked to give a presentation, and instead of using the knowledge and experience you already have, you feel you need to learn more. You spend hours researching additional data, reading more articles, and gathering resources, yet you still don't feel ready. As the presentation date approaches, you're overwhelmed by the idea that you haven't learnt enough, even though you're already an expert on the subject.

Home example: you're tackling a home renovation project, and instead of asking for help or hiring a professional, you dive into researching every possible detail about materials, design options, and techniques. You spend hours watching DIY videos and reading articles, determined to become an expert in every aspect of the project. You feel anxious about making a mistake or not knowing enough, so you avoid asking for advice, thinking that if you don't handle it perfectly yourself, you'll look inexperienced or unqualified. Even when someone offers to help, you hesitate because you're convinced that they won't do it "the right way".

Not sure if this applies to you? Ask yourself:

- Do you spend excessive time gathering information, even when you already have what you need to move forward?
- Do you feel like you can't take action until you know everything, even though you're capable of learning as you go?

4. Must do it alone

You feel that asking for help means you're not strong enough or capable enough. This belief makes it hard to collaborate with others, even when teamwork could make the job easier. You struggle with delegating, believing that you should handle everything yourself, which can lead to unnecessary stress and isolation.

Work example: you're given a project that requires collaboration, but you refuse to ask for help. You think that asking for assistance would make you seem incapable, so you try to do everything yourself. In the end, you're overwhelmed, the quality of your work suffers, and you feel frustrated because you didn't reach out when you had the opportunity to share the load.

Home example: you're trying to juggle all the household chores – cleaning, organizing, grocery shopping, and managing your family's admin and diary. Even when you're feeling overwhelmed, you hesitate to ask anyone for help because you believe that doing it all yourself is the only way to prove you're capable. You might even refuse to let your partner or children pitch in, thinking that if they take over any task, it somehow reflects poorly on you. You worry that if others step in, they'll see you as incompetent or not doing your part. So you push through, stressing over every detail, just to prove that you can manage everything on your own. This is a delegation-free zone.

Not sure if this applies to you? Ask yourself:

- Do you feel like asking for help means you're not strong enough or capable enough?
- Do you avoid delegating tasks, even when it would make your life easier?

Activity: Your Imposter: Spot It, Face It, Send it Packing

Now that you've explored the different ways impostorism can show up, it's time to identify which one resonates most with you and create an action plan for change. The good news is, we're not powerless in the face of impostor feelings. Yes, they're a normal part of life, but we can definitely learn to recognize them, resist them, and minimize their impact. There's no reason why this self-doubt should hold us back from pursuing our purpose. I'll offer some questions to reflect on in your journal and suggest a few steps you can take, but I also encourage you to think of your own solutions. After all, you know yourself better than I do – plus, I don't want to do *all* the heavy lifting!

- Which impostor type do you most resonate with? There will probably be more than one but do try to narrow it down.

- What is one area of your life (work, home, relationships) where you're feeling most like an impostor right now? Why?
- What aspects of your personality (think about the work we did in Chapters 2, 3, and 4) are helping, and which are hindering your progress in this area?
- When you think about your purpose, does self-doubt ever stand in the way of pursuing it?

Now you've identified your impostorism type and how it is holding you back, it's time to think about how to overcome this. For each type, I've provided some reflection, an affirmation (which would be good to build into your daily practice), and then a suggested action for you to use as a starting point.

For the Must Be Perfect

- **Reflect:** what would happen if you allowed yourself to make mistakes and learn from them? What does "good enough" look like for you, and where can you begin to embrace it?
- **Affirmation:** I embrace progress over perfection. I trust in my ability to grow through mistakes and celebrate the lessons they bring.
- **Action:** try setting small, manageable goals where "done is better than perfect". Celebrate progress instead of perfection.

For the Must Juggle It All

- **Reflect:** is there a pattern where, even when you're overloaded, you keep saying yes to more tasks or commitments? Do you expect others to manage as much as you do? Why is rest not allowed for you?
- **Affirmation:** I am worthy of rest and balance. My value isn't measured by how much I do, but by who I am.
- **Action:** use time-blocking techniques to help you focus on

one task at a time, without feeling the need to multitask. This can help reduce the sense of overwhelm. Add a block in for rest.

For the Must Know It All

- **Reflect:** how can you embrace the idea that learning is a lifelong process, and no one knows everything? What would it feel like to know less than others in the room and be comfortable about it? How can you share your unique experiences and viewpoint rather than always relying on knowledge?
- **Affirmation:** I am constantly learning, and I embrace the beauty of not knowing everything. Every step of growth is valuable, and I have the courage to seek knowledge and share it with others.
- **Action:** recognize there will be more questions than you can answer, and approach challenges with curiosity rather than the need for immediate answers. Start practising just-in-time learning, or setting a time limit for how long you can spend learning for any given task, acknowledging you will never know it all.

For the Must Do It Alone

- **Reflect:** how would it feel to ask for help or accept support from others without feeling like you're losing your independence? Do you expect others to operate without help and support? Why do you feel that help isn't something that you should receive?
- **Affirmation:** I am strong enough to ask for support when I need it. Collaborating with others enriches my life and helps me fulfil my purpose with greater ease and connection.
- **Action:** ask for help on something small this week, whether it's at work or home, and notice how it changes the experience for you.

Self-Sabotaging Behaviour 2: Fixed Mindset

I don't like heights, and I'm sure I've got worse as I've got older. I'm okay in a plane (just about), and I'm fine when I'm on a zip wire if I know the ground isn't too far away. But bridges? Not so much. And steep cliff edges, where I might fall off – that's a whole different story. But I have three sons who, along with their dad, seem to have no fear whatsoever. On a recent holiday, we visited a high rope course like no other I have ever experienced. The boys wanted to push on and tackle the most difficult routes – levels 9 and 10. I had little energy left but felt an overwhelming need to keep up, for reasons I couldn't quite understand (and still don't). Level 9 used every last ounce of my physical and emotional strength to complete – a 250-metre (over 800 feet) zip wire from some rather precarious ledges. When I finally finished, I felt a huge sense of relief and accomplishment, but the torture wasn't yet over.

We moved on to level 10, which we'd been told was easier than level 9. It wasn't. I only realized this halfway through, with no easy way down except to continue. I had to scale the side of an actual bridge, climb over it, and then zip wire down. The trouble was, by this point I was completely drained and had no reserves to draw from. I was so close, yet so far. My knees were knocking, my eyes were watering, and that all too familiar voice in my head was saying:

"I can't do it."

My hands were sweaty, clinging on for dear life, and my body was exhausted. But one tentative step at a time, with a little help from my friends, I completed that final course. Genuinely, tears of sheer relief rolled down my sweaty face, and I felt a modicum of pride.

I couldn't do it – and yet, somehow, I did.

How often do you hold back from new opportunities because you fear you won't be able to succeed? How often do you discount yourself from a new job because you can't tick every box on the list? How often do you hesitate to take on a challenge simply because you might fail? This is called having a fixed mindset.

Fixed and Growth Mindsets

You may have heard the phrase "fixed or growth mindset" thrown around, but it's often misunderstood and misapplied as a tool to push people into doing things they don't want to do or aren't really wired to do. In reality it's best seen as a framework for understanding how we approach obstacles, challenges, and opportunities – and recognizing how we often stand in the way of our own growth and purpose. It's difficult to move towards the life you've been searching for with the fear of failure holding you back.

The concept of fixed and growth mindsets stems from the life's work of Carol Dweck, an American psychologist whose inspiration came from her own experiences in primary school. She observed how many people, including herself, viewed intelligence as an innate, fixed trait. Able pupils often avoided challenges for fear of failure, reluctant to risk revealing that their so-called talents and abilities might have limits. Rather than embracing the opportunity to grow through harder work, they chose instead to coast, avoiding situations where they might falter, and inadvertently stunting their potential in the process.

A growth mindset is the belief that abilities can be developed through effort, learning, and perseverance. In contrast, a fixed mindset assumes that our abilities are set in stone and unable to change.[5] Those with a fixed mindset often approach learning with the aim of appearing smart, avoiding challenges for fear that hard work or mistakes might reveal a lack of innate ability. On the other hand, individuals with a growth mindset view effort as a key driver of progress and see setbacks not as failures, but as opportunities to develop new skills and improve. This perspective encourages resilience, adaptability, and a willingness to embrace challenges as part of the journey towards growth.

There are a few more pointers we need to understand, to avoid misusing this important research in our own lives and beating ourselves up whenever we have a wobble about stepping out or trying challenging things.

Everyone has both mindsets

Nobody has a 100 per cent growth mindset all the time, and neither is this a realistic goal. The aim is to recognize the impact of our thinking and then choose to do differently when we sense we are retreating, avoiding failure, or giving up too soon. As Carol puts it, "Everyone is actually a mixture of fixed and growth mindsets, and that mixture continually evolves with experience. A pure growth mindset doesn't exist, which we must acknowledge to attain the benefits we seek."[6]

It's not about ignoring your personality

It would be easy to assume that adopting a growth mindset means striving to improve at everything and anything, without any strategy or focus. But as adults, we have a limited amount of time on Earth to grow, develop, and pursue our purpose, so we need to focus our efforts with intention on the things that matter most. If we aimlessly try and get better at everything, we risk diluting our efforts and compromising our level of competence in areas where we truly excel – our true strengths. By focusing on what aligns with our personality, passions, and talents, we can grow in ways that are both impactful and purposeful.

It's all about effort and practice

The underlying message of growth mindsets isn't a simplistic, "You can be or do anything you want to". Instead, it's a recognition that anything that's truly worth pursuing – anything meaningful or rewarding – requires effort, stamina, perseverance, and practice. Success is rarely, if ever, the product of innate talent alone. There will always come a point where natural abilities meet their limit.

That's often where people with a fixed mindset stop, believing that if something doesn't come easily, they're simply not capable.

However, a growth mindset reframes this challenge. It's at this very point – when natural talent falls short – that effort, practice, and resilience take centre stage. Those with a growth mindset understand that skills and abilities aren't fixed but can be developed with dedication and hard work. This mindset allows us to see setbacks as opportunities to improve rather than insurmountable barriers. It shifts the focus from a fear of failure to the possibility of growth, unlocking the determination to push through discomfort and take us further than we ever thought possible.

This perspective doesn't just lead to better results; it also builds character, deepens self-belief, and brings us closer to a life of purpose. By embracing challenges as part of the journey, we open the door to achieving things we might have once thought impossible.

Failure isn't a personality trait

One of the most powerful aspects of Carol Dweck's work is her perspective on failure. She challenges us to stop seeing failure as a reflection of our identity and instead view it as a natural part of growth; something that happens to anyone striving to improve. Think about a time in your life when you experienced a significant leap forward. Chances are it involved some kind of failure: losing a job or opportunity, a project that went wrong, or even failing an important exam. These moments demand that we step up, adapt, and grow.

Yet, many of us devote an extraordinary amount of energy to avoiding even the possibility of failure. But here's the truth: you are not defined by what you do, nor by what you fail at. Michael Jordan, arguably one of the greatest basketball players of all time, famously embraced his failures. In a Nike ad, he reflected: "I've missed more than 9,000 shots in my career. I've lost almost 300 games. Twenty-six times I've been trusted to take the game-winning shot and missed. I've failed over and over and over again in my life. And that is why I succeed." [7]

If someone like Michael Jordan can own his failures and credit them for his success, why shouldn't we? Failure is not the opposite of success – it's a stepping stone towards it.

So, in principle we get it. Our talents can be developed, hard doesn't mean we're rubbish, and practice makes progress. But knowing this isn't always enough. How do we stop ourselves from holding back, playing it safe, and metaphorically keeping our hand down in class? How do we push past the fear of getting it wrong or not being good enough?

- **Add "yet" to your vocabulary**: whenever you find yourself saying that you can't do something, simply add the word "yet". It's a powerful word that shifts the emphasis of your sentence. The word "yet" signals that your abilities are not fixed and reminds you that growth is a process. It's a case of "fake it 'til you make it" – you don't have to believe it, yet, but by beginning to speak it, we change the narrative.
- **Change your goals**: if you're noticing that all your goals are outcome driven, think about how you can reword them to be process or learning driven instead. For example, instead of aiming to "get the promotion", focus on "developing leadership skills" or "mastering key aspects of the role". Learning goals create room for mistakes and progress, which are essential for developing a growth mindset.
- **Go for 1% "microshifts"**: if there's an area of your natural talent and true strengths that you want to develop, ask yourself, "What does it look like if I do that 1% better every day?" What's a doable "microshift" that over time adds up to real change and development in your life? For example, if I

love learning and want to know more about something that is interesting to me, 1% better might be agreeing to read about it for 10 minutes every day.

Make Mistakes

This is definitely a work in progress for me, but I've come to realize that if I'm not making any mistakes, I'm probably not growing. As much as I'd prefer to avoid them, I'm learning to embrace mistakes and treat them as opportunities to learn and improve.

I recently heard a brilliant story that perfectly captures this idea. A waiter in a high-end restaurant accidentally served some very lucky diners a £4,500 bottle of wine instead of the £260 bottle they'd ordered. Naturally, the staff member was mortified (though the diners were likely overjoyed), and you'd be forgiven for thinking this was grounds for immediate dismissal. But the restaurant chose to handle the mistake with grace and humanity, turning the situation into a masterclass in leadership and culture.

They took to Twitter with a post that went viral:

> *"To the customer who accidentally got given a bottle of Château Le Pin Pomerol 2001, which is £4,500 on our menu, last night – hope you enjoyed your evening! To the member of staff who accidentally gave it away, chin up! One-off mistakes happen, and we love you anyway."*[8]

The response was overwhelmingly positive, with praise pouring in from all over the world. The restaurant saw a surge in bookings, as people flocked for a chance to experience the kind of establishment that values its people so highly. And that waiter? I bet they'll never make the same mistake again!

Mistakes aren't easy to face, but what truly matters is how we respond to them. They can be powerful moments for growth, reflection, and resilience – if we let them.

Coaching Notes: Priya's Story

Priya sought coaching because she felt stuck in her career, unsure whether to push forward or walk away. Deep down, she recognized a pattern of self-sabotage holding her back. A few years into her legal career, early mistakes and a lack of support had left her second-guessing every decision. Rather than asking for help – fearing it would make her look incompetent – Priya tried to shoulder everything alone, desperately striving to get it right.

Adding to her struggles, Priya felt out of place. Having spent much of her childhood overseas, her early years in the UK had been tough, leaving her feeling like she didn't fully belong. Although Priya was confident and ambitious in many respects, she often overcompensated for her perceived differences. She pushed herself relentlessly, crafting the image of someone who had it all together – like a graceful swan gliding on the surface, masking the frantic paddling beneath.

This façade was taking its toll, draining her peace of mind, straining her relationships, and eroding her confidence. Priya questioned whether she even deserved her role, convinced it was only a matter of time before everyone discovered she wasn't as capable as they thought. She equated not knowing something with incompetence, rather than as an opportunity to learn and grow.

Priya was caught in the double bind of a fixed mindset as well as impostorism – a powerful combination that left her paralyzed and doubting her worth.

In our session, Priya reacquainted herself with her true strengths, those parts of her personality that made her a brilliant lawyer: what she was best placed to do, what she needed to do more of, and what she needed to do less of. We focused on her excellent relationship-building skills, and how she could lean into these to find some excellent mentorship, finding places she could practise asking for help and learn to make mistakes more safely. Priya also recognized that her early experiences are what gave her a beautiful difference, a way of connecting with others, and an understanding of being the "new girl", and so offered her services as a mentor for the new graduates joining the team. Priya may want a new career challenge one day, but she's recognized that for now, the work she needed to do was on her perspective, recognizing that none of us has all that we need, and that making mistakes and asking for help make for better outcomes.

Activity: Shift Your Mindset

Here's a reflective activity idea to help you move from a fixed to a growth mindset. The purpose is to help you identify areas in your life where a fixed mindset might be holding you back and to reframe your approach to challenges, mistakes, and growth opportunities. You might want to get out that journal.

Step 1: Spot the fixed mindset

Think of a recent situation where you hesitated, avoided, or gave up on something because you feared failure or doubted your abilities. Reflect on these questions:

- What was the challenge?
- What thoughts or feelings did you experience? For example, "I'm not good at this", "I'll look foolish if I fail".
- How did this affect your actions or decisions?

Write down one or two examples, and be honest with yourself.

Step 2: Reframe the narrative

Using the examples you just wrote, rewrite the story from a growth mindset perspective. For each scenario:

- What could you tell yourself instead of the fixed mindset thoughts? For example, "I'm not good at this *yet*", or "I can learn from this experience".
- How can your natural personality give you a fresh perspective on how you could succeed in this area? Think about your natural strengths and talents and decide how they can help you grow.
- What small step could you take to move forward, even if it feels challenging?
- How might failure in this situation help you grow or learn something new?

Example:

- Fixed mindset thought: I can't present in front of a large group because I'm terrible at public speaking.
- Growth mindset reframe: public speaking is a skill I can improve with practice. Every attempt makes me better.
- Personality perspective: I can use my attention to detail to work hard on rehearsing the content, or I can use my relationship-building strengths to connect with the audience.
- Action step: volunteer to give a short update in the next team meeting.

Step 3: Practise the power of "yet"

Reflect on areas in your life where you've thought, "I can't do this". Write down three "I can't" statements and add the word "yet" to the end of each. For example:

- I can't manage a large team... yet
- I can't run a 5K... yet
- I can't speak a new language fluently... yet

Notice how the word "yet" shifts your mindset towards possibility and growth.

Step 4: Identify your microshift

Growth happens one small step at a time. Choose one area where you'd like to develop and identify a 1% improvement you can commit to daily or weekly (using your unique strengths and personality to help you).

- What is one area of your life where you'd like to develop?
- What is one small, actionable habit or practice you can start today?
- How will you track your progress?

Step 5: Redefine failure

Reflect on a time when you made a mistake or failed at something. Ask yourself:

- What did I learn from this experience?
- How did this failure help me grow, even if it didn't feel like it at the time?
- How might I approach a similar situation differently in the future, and how can I use my strengths to help me?

Bonus tip: next time you make a mistake, or miss out on an opportunity, write a note in your diary as a reminder that it happened, but jot it on a date about six months *after* the event took place. Then, when you come across the reminder in the future, it will help you realize it was less important than you originally thought, or even acted as the catalyst for your growth.

Self-Sabotaging Behaviour 3: Set Yourself Free From Comparison

A few years ago, I was invited to be a main stage speaker at a conference. It was a bigger opportunity than I was used to, but I had made a promise to myself that year to say yes to anything that scared me a little. So, I said yes.

As the event drew closer, the publicity started rolling out on social media. And there, alongside my name, was the name of a hugely respected speaker – someone at the very top of their field. They were a master of their craft, with far more experience and credibility than me. Their name was right next to mine.

I felt sick.

To make matters worse, friends excitedly sent me screenshots of the promo posts, our headshots side by side. But instead of feeling proud, I spiralled into comparison. This wasn't just impostor syndrome: I was measuring myself directly against someone I *knew* was better. How could I follow them? How could I stand on the same stage? I just wasn't as good as they were.

So many times on social media I've seen people thriving in the field I want to be in – landing dream clients, signing book deals, and winning awards. And instead of just feeling happy for them, I've found myself comparing and thinking, "Why not me? Why am I not getting those opportunities?"

And it's not just work. Over the years, I've compared everything – people's situations, families, friendships, holidays, appearances. You name it, I've probably measured myself against it.

And then there have been other moments – the ones I'm most reluctant to admit. The times when I've compared myself, my life, or what I own to someone else's, and – at least in my own mind – I've come out on top. These moments don't leave me with a sense of lack or jealousy like the others do. Instead, they leave me with a different kind of discomfort, one that feels even worse: smugness.

It's that fleeting, self-satisfied feeling of "at least I'm doing better than them" – a thought I'm not proud of, but one that has crossed my mind more times than I'd like to admit. And the truth is, this kind of comparison is just as toxic. Because whether I'm putting myself above or below someone else, I'm still measuring my worth in relation to theirs. And I know I'm not the only one.

So, why do we do it? Why do we constantly compare ourselves to others? Well, we're actually wired to. As human beings, we have an innate drive to understand ourselves. This capacity for self-reflection is one of the defining traits of our species. It's what makes us look up at the stars and question our purpose, keeps us from behaving like freshers at the office Christmas party, and fuels our instinct to compete with those around us.

This peculiar drive was first explored in depth by social psychologist Leon Festinger in 1954.[9] He proposed the Social Comparison Theory, which suggests that we compare ourselves to others for two main reasons:

- To reduce uncertainty about where we stand in different areas of life.
- To define ourselves, shaping our self-concept based on how we measure up to those around us.

According to Festinger, we don't define ourselves in a vacuum – we do it in relation to others. And interestingly, we're more likely to compare ourselves to people who are similar to us in ways we find important. This means we're more inclined to measure ourselves against a colleague at our level rather than the CEO, or to compare our running times with someone in our weekly running group rather than Usain Bolt. The bigger the gap between us and another person, the less relevant the comparison feels.

Festinger identified two types of social comparison:

- **Upward comparison** happens when we compare ourselves to someone who seems to be in a better position – more successful, more skilled, or more accomplished. This can sometimes be motivating, but more often than not it leads to feelings of inadequacy or jealousy.
- **Downward comparison** happens when we compare ourselves to someone worse off, giving us a temporary self-esteem boost. But let's be honest: while chasing this feeling might seem satisfying in the moment, it never really lasts. Using other people's shortcomings as a foundation for self-worth is flimsy at best. Because sooner or later you'll encounter someone who outshines you, and the cycle starts all over again.

You may have heard the saying, "Comparison is the thief of joy." Never has a truer word been spoken, but I'd take it even further. Comparison doesn't just steal our joy; it directly impacts our self-esteem and robs us of our sense of purpose. When we're constantly measuring our lives against others, we lose sight of our own unique path – our goals, values, and the things that truly matter to us. Instead of focusing on what drives us and brings us fulfilment, we get caught in an endless cycle of trying to measure up, leaving us disconnected from the things that give our lives meaning. And now, thanks to social media, we're no longer measuring ourselves against just a handful of people, we're comparing ourselves to the entire world. And it's taking a serious toll on our wellbeing. One study found that after a year or more of using Facebook, people tend to perceive others as happier and view life as unfair. Another study demonstrated that individuals interacting with strangers on the platform (in other words, accounts beyond personal connections) were more likely to believe that others on the platform had better lives than they did.[10]

Additionally, research reveals that people often underestimate others' negative emotions, leading to "emotional pluralistic ignorance", which is the mistaken belief that they are alone in their struggles. This happens because individuals tend to present themselves as happier than they truly are, which can deepen feelings of loneliness and isolation for those facing emotional difficulties.[11] Is the grass greener on the other side? Or is it just fake grass?

Perhaps the grass is greener where you water it.

A Different Way

If we can accept that comparison is inevitable for most of us, how can we reframe it so that it doesn't hold us back? The good news is there's a way to shift our perspective.

There's a wise saying I usually come back to, often attributed to Martin Luther: "You cannot keep birds from flying over your head, but you can keep them from building a nest in your hair." In other words, we can't always stop those initial thoughts of comparison – whether they leave us feeling inadequate or inflated – but we *can* choose what happens next. We don't need to let that thought pull up a chair and make itself at home in our heads.

Here are five ways to take control of comparison before it takes control of you.

1: Choose celebration over comparison

The next time you see someone doing or having something you wish for yourself, choose to be happy for them. You don't even have to feel it at first, just practise saying, "Good for them", and keep repeating it until you start to mean it. Gratitude and celebration can become habits, just like comparison can.

2: Reject the scarcity mindset

It's easy to slip into the belief that there's only a limited supply of good things in the world – that if someone else gets an opportunity, it somehow reduces your chances. But success isn't a pie with only so many slices. Just because something great happens for someone else doesn't mean there's less available for you. There is enough to go around.

3: Use good news as motivation

Instead of seeing someone else's success as a reason to feel discouraged, use it as proof that good things are possible. Let it inspire you as to what could be for you, too. I have a friend who struggled to conceive for years, and instead of letting pregnancy announcements bring her down, she used them as reminders that it *could* happen for her, too. She chose hope over comparison.

4: Be mindful of how you measure your worth

If your self-worth is built on feeling better than others, it's on shaky ground, because there will always be someone ahead of you and someone behind you. Avoid building your security on something that can be taken from you at any moment. Instead of using comparison to feel superior, pause and shift your focus to gratitude. What is good in *your* life right now?

5: Remember that highlight reels don't tell the full story

Social media is filled with curated snapshots – engagement announcements, career wins, trips of a lifetime – but for every moment of joy someone shares, there are unseen struggles, disappointments, and challenges. As one wise person put it: "The reason we struggle with insecurity is because we compare our behind-the-scenes with everyone else's highlight reel." The next time social media leaves you feeling less-than, remind yourself of this truth: nobody's life is perfect all the time. Everyone has more going on than we realize. Celebrate their wins, but don't assume you know their full story.

One last thought on social media: if we're sometimes impacted by what others post, it's likely our own posts affect people, too.

This is something I try to be mindful of, finding a balance between celebrating the good and acknowledging the everyday realities. I don't want someone to look at my life and feel a sense of lack. A helpful practice is to pause and ask ourselves, "Why am I sharing this? What outcome am I hoping for? Do my intentions align with my values?" A little self-awareness can go a long way in creating a more authentic and considerate online space.

Stay in Your Lane

When I say, "stay in your lane", it's not intended as a put-down. I don't mean shrink yourself or avoid growth. I don't mean play it small or refuse to dream big. I don't mean mind your own business and stick to what you know. What I do mean is this: you have a unique lane to walk, one that fits your strengths, talents, personality, and purpose. And the more time you spend fixating on someone else's journey, the less time you have to cultivate your own.

If I spend my life staring at your lane, at all the great things happening for you, I risk missing out on the opportunities and strengths I might encounter. But when I focus on my own path, lean into who I am, and plan out my own journey, I create a life that's purposeful for me and those around me. So, when you catch yourself comparing, come back to this truth: nobody can do what you do quite the way you do it. Your contribution is unique and incomparable.

Back to my story of being a mainstage speaker alongside someone far more experienced than me. I had a choice to make: spend my preparation time obsessing over how I wasn't as polished, compelling, or accomplished as them, or focus on showing up as the best version of me. With a little help from my friends, I chose the second option.

First, I decided to redefine my measure of success. If success meant "being better than him", I was almost guaranteed to fall short. So instead, I decided success would be measured by how well I prepared and how fully I showed up as me.

I made a list of what makes me a good speaker: honesty, storytelling, and practicality. And I intentionally leaned into those strengths. On the day of the event, I listened to him speak first. He was brilliant. But instead of letting that intimidate me, I appreciated his work and recognized how different it was from my own. Both styles could be valuable at the same time; no comparison needed.

I stayed in my lane, and I think I did a pretty good job of it.

Activity: Embrace Your Lane

Comparison is natural, but it doesn't have to define you. Take a moment to reflect on the ideas in this chapter and how they apply to your own life. You might want to take some notes in your journal.

Step 1: Notice your patterns

Think about the last time you found yourself caught in comparison, whether it left you feeling inadequate or superior. Write down:

- Who or what you were comparing yourself to, and what were the triggers
- How it made you feel
- What thoughts ran through your mind

Step 2: Reframe the comparison

Now, rewrite the experience through a new lens:

- If you felt inadequate, how can you shift towards celebration or motivation?
- If you felt superior, how can you re-centre on gratitude rather than comparison?
- Who in your life can you appreciate and celebrate for their strengths and talents instead of comparing yourself to them?

- What truth can you remind yourself of that keeps you grounded in your own journey?
- Are there any self-destructive habits that you might need to stop doing? (For example, unfollow certain social media accounts)

Step 3: Your unique contribution

Comparison distracts us from our own strengths. Instead of focusing on what others are doing, take a moment to celebrate *your* lane.

- What are three qualities that make you uniquely you? (Think about the work you have already done on this)
- What are three strengths or talents you bring to the table?
- How can you lean into these in your work, relationships, or personal growth, especially the next time you're triggered to compare?

Step 4: Set an intention

As you move forward, how can you break the cycle of comparison? Choose one action to focus on this week:

- Choose celebration over comparison; practise saying, "Good for them" when you see someone succeeding
- Reject the scarcity mindset and remind yourself there is enough to go around
- Use good news as motivation and let someone else's success inspire you rather than discourage you
- Be mindful of your self-worth and shift from comparison to gratitude
- Curate your social media experience: pause before posting or consuming content and ask, "Why am I sharing this?"

Write down your chosen action and keep it somewhere visible. The more intentional you are about where you focus your energy, the more you'll grow in confidence and purpose.

Self-Sabotaging Behaviour 4: People Pleasing

How often do you find yourself agreeing to things you don't want to do, just to keep the peace? Holding back from disagreeing with a colleague, even when you strongly feel otherwise? Taking on yet another Parent-Teacher Association task despite already being overwhelmed? Saying yes to plans when you'd rather stay home? Insisting you don't mind when, deep down, you do? If the answer to some or all of these questions is "a lot", you might just be a people pleaser.

People pleasing is more than just wanting to please other people, because there's nothing intrinsically wrong with wanting to do that. It's when our decisions and behaviours regularly, even systematically, put the needs of others above our own. People pleasers can be kind, agreeable, generous, and helpful, but they have trouble advocating for themselves, which then means that these kind behaviours lead to a harmful level of self-sacrifice or even self-neglect. There's a fine line between being a supportive friend, a team player, and an eager volunteer, and saying yes to everything at the expense of your own wellbeing or reputation. People pleasing happens when we tip dangerously from healthy generosity into self-sacrifice. Author and self-advocacy coach Hailey Magee hits the nail on the head: "When we're people pleasing, our insides don't match our outsides."[12] When we're being genuinely kind, we help others because we want to; it feels good and aligns with our values. But when kindness stems from people pleasing, we may appear easy-going and agreeable on the outside while feeling resentful, overwhelmed, or exhausted on the inside. That inner conflict is the clearest sign that our generosity has crossed into people-pleasing territory.

It's less about the behaviour itself, but the motivation behind it. Is your "yes" driven by a need for acceptance, validation, or fear of rejection? Or is it freely given, without resentment, as a genuine act of generosity? And this matters, because people pleasing takes a toll on our health and wellbeing and rarely leads to positive long-term outcomes for anyone involved. People pleasing reinforces the belief that we're not good enough, blocks genuine connections, and leads us to neglect our own needs. We suppress our emotions and opinions, teach people to treat us in ways that don't honour us, and ultimately operate from a place of dishonesty, and even manipulation. Beyond this, people pleasing robs us of the chance to pursue our own purpose. We're so busy chasing what others want for us that we have no space to go after what's truly best for us.

Identifying Behaviour Patterns

Recognizing our true motivations isn't always easy; it takes time and effort to step back and identify patterns of behaviour for what they really are. So, let's explore some specific ways people pleasing can show up in our lives, and what lies at the root of it.

You're overwhelmed but unwilling to express your needs

Your plate is not just full, it's overflowing, yet you continue to take on more. At work, you say yes to extra projects and responsibilities, stepping in to fill the gaps left by others. At home, you shoulder additional tasks, and with friends or volunteer commitments, you keep agreeing to help despite having no time to spare. The problem is that you struggle to voice how overwhelmed you feel. Saying no or advocating for yourself feels daunting, and the thought of potential conflict is even harder to bear. So, you push through, taking on more and more until the weight of responsibility is matched only by a growing sense of resentment.

You're overwhelmed but still strive for perfection

You're juggling more than you can handle, yet you hold yourself to impossibly high standards. Every task must be done flawlessly: at work, at home, and in your personal commitments. You double-check, refine, and push yourself to go the extra mile, even when time and energy are in short supply. Everything you do must be outstanding. Mistakes feel unacceptable, and the thought of letting someone down is unbearable. Instead of easing up, you push harder, convincing yourself that if you just try a little more, you'll keep everything under control. But the pressure is relentless, and exhaustion and frustration build beneath the surface. No matter how much you achieve, it never quite feels enough.

You're overwhelmed but feel obligated to meet others' expectations

You're stretched thin, yet the expectations placed on you – by family, friends, work, and even society – keep pulling you in every direction. Your family relies on you, your friends count on you, and your workplace expects you to step up. There's an unspoken pressure to be reliable, capable, and always available. Beyond that, societal expectations whisper that you should be achieving more, giving more, and balancing it all with grace. The weight of these demands makes it hard to say no, even when you're already at your limit. Everyone else is doing it, so why not you? So you keep showing up, meeting obligations, and fulfilling roles until the pressure becomes overwhelming. And while you do it all for others, deep down you wonder if there's any space left for yourself.

You're overwhelmed but this is how you feel validated and accepted

You're overwhelmed, yet if you're honest, a part of you thrives on being needed. Saying yes, stepping up, and pushing through exhaustion isn't just about responsibility, it's how you feel valued.

Accomplishing more, helping others, and meeting expectations bring a sense of purpose – even when it comes at your own expense. You fear that slowing down or setting boundaries might make you seem less capable, less dependable, or even less worthy. So you keep going, seeking validation through productivity and self-sacrifice. But no matter how much you give, the feeling of being enough remains just out of reach, leaving you caught between exhaustion and the need for approval.

You may find yourself relating to one, or even all, of these patterns. Recognizing what drives our behaviour is the first step towards change.

The Personality Factor

As we explored in Chapter 5, our greatest strengths and talents can sometimes work against us. The very qualities that define us can also trip us up if we're not mindful. People pleasing is a universal challenge and affects all personality types in different ways.

Consider your own personality: what aspects of it make you more prone to people pleasing? For example, I know that I'm naturally open, warm, and genuinely like most people I meet. As a result, I want to be liked in return. Enter people pleasing: "I'll do what you ask because I want your approval and fear rejection." Is that entirely bad? Not at all. Can it become a problem? Absolutely.

Here's another example. If you're a natural peacemaker, you excel at creating harmony and helping people work well together, eliminating tension and stress. But that same strength can fuel people pleasing: "I'll agree to this because I'd rather inconvenience myself than risk conflict or an uncomfortable conversation."

Back in Chapter 2, you identified which strength type you align with most. Now, let's explore how people pleasing might show up within each of those types.

The Achiever

How you might people please:

- Saying yes to too many commitments because you want to be seen as dependable and competent
- Taking on more work than necessary to maintain your reputation as a high performer
- Struggling to delegate because you feel responsible for results, even at the cost of your wellbeing
- Equating your self-worth with productivity, leading you to overextend to gain approval

The Thinker

How you might people please:

- Over-explaining or justifying your thoughts to ensure others understand them fully
- Struggling to say no to giving advice, feeling responsible for helping others work things out
- Avoiding confrontation by staying in analysis mode rather than asserting your own needs
- Refraining from taking risks or making decisions for fear of disappointing others with the outcome

The Connector

How you might people please:

- Prioritizing others' emotional needs at the expense of your own wellbeing
- Saying yes to social obligations to avoid disappointing or upsetting anyone
- Avoiding necessary conflict to keep the peace, even when you should set boundaries
- Feeling guilty for putting yourself first, fearing you'll let people down

The Impactor

How you might people please:

- Taking on too much responsibility for others' success, believing you must lead and inspire at all times
- Feeling pressure to constantly perform or be "on", fearing you might lose influence if you show vulnerability
- Saying yes to opportunities just to maintain your leadership role, even if they don't align with your values
- Struggling to accept constructive feedback without seeing it as a personal failure

The Believer

How you might people please:

- Feeling obligated to help when you see someone struggling, even at personal cost
- Avoiding saying no to causes or commitments because you feel a deep sense of duty
- Feeling responsible for guiding others towards what's "right", even when it drains you
- Struggling to prioritize yourself, believing self-care is selfish when others need you

The Explorer

How you might people please:

- Saying yes to too many new opportunities to avoid missing out or disappointing others, regardless of whether it's the best fit for you
- Struggling with commitment, fearing that saying no to one thing will close doors forever
- Constantly shifting focus to keep others engaged, rather than staying true to your own path

- Avoiding deep confrontation or difficult discussions in favour of staying "light and fun"

How to Stop People Pleasing

Here's my controversial opinion: I don't think we *should* stop people pleasing. Yes, we need to get it under control. Yes, we need to set boundaries. But should we stop putting ourselves out, going the extra mile, or doing things we don't necessarily want to? I don't think so. So much advice out there tells us to put ourselves first, say no to anything that doesn't directly serve us, and build a life that revolves entirely around our own needs, regardless of what anyone else thinks. But this approach has flaws.

First, as you're reading this, you likely want a life of purpose – one that's good for you, your loved ones, and the world around you. Completely disregarding others just isn't who you are. You care, and you *want* to care. Telling you to stop prioritizing the needs of others doesn't align with your core values.

Second, research shows that acts of generosity – helping others without expecting anything in return – lead to greater purpose, happiness, and even better physical and mental health. Givers tend to live longer and have a higher quality of life. However, there's a key distinction: these benefits only apply when the act of giving is a *choice*, not something done out of fear, obligation, or a desire for approval.[13]

And here we come to the crux of the issue: choice. True generosity comes from a place of freedom, not from anxiety, low self-worth, or a fear of disappointing others. So, instead of stopping people pleasing altogether, the goal is to know when to say yes and when to say no; when to put yourself out there and when to protect your time and energy. Here are some practical strategies to help you stay true to who you are, while building in the boundaries you need.

Give yourself time to think

Release yourself from the feeling that you need to give an immediate answer: most requests just aren't as urgent as they seem. Instead of feeling pressured to respond on the spot, practise pausing. A simple response like, "Let me check my diary and get back to you", or "I need a little time to think about that", creates that bit of space to stop and consider whether saying yes aligns with your priorities and capacity. This small habit helps you move away from automatic, knee-jerk agreements and ensures that when you do say yes, it's intentional and genuine rather than driven by obligation.

Avoid the "busy" competition

One challenge in setting boundaries or saying no is the urge to justify our decision by proving just how busy we are. This problem is a bit of a hybrid between people pleasing and comparison behaviour. We fall into the trap of listing our overflowing responsibilities, as if our only right to decline comes from being completely maxed out. But this mindset fuels unhelpful comparisons and reinforces the toxic hustle culture that equates our worth with our level of busyness. Instead of measuring your value by how much you can juggle, step off the "busy train" and define your own internal metrics, ones that prioritize your peace and alignment over exhaustion.

I once heard someone gracefully decline a request by saying, "My plate is as full as I'd like it to be right now," and I love that. No competitive comparison, no need to prove they were busier than anyone else. Just a simple, self-assured recognition of their limits. That's the kind of boundary-setting that truly empowers us.

Set pre-decided limits

Saying no, or yes for that matter, becomes much easier when you've already decided in advance what your ideal schedule and commitments look like. Having clear personal boundaries helps you filter requests without hesitation or guilt. For example, when our boys were younger, we made a family rule: unless there was something truly exceptional, we would keep either Friday or Saturday night reserved for family time. This wasn't up for negotiation because we knew it created the rhythm that felt right for us. So, when invitations for dinner or other events came in, we had a built-in decision-making framework. If saying yes meant losing both weekend nights together, the answer was a simple and confident no.

You can create similar parameters in your own life. How many evenings a week do you want to be out? How many extracurricular activities can you realistically juggle? How many volunteer hours fit into your schedule? What childcare arrangement feels right for your family? Setting these guidelines in advance helps you make decisions that align with your values rather than defaulting to people pleasing.

It goes without saying that you don't need to be rigid about this – there are times and seasons to bend out of shape. But for the most part, having pre-agreed limits allows you to purposefully protect your time and energy.

Ask yourself this question

This question has genuinely transformed how I approach requests for my time and help. Before taking on anything new, pause and ask yourself, "If I say yes to this, what am I saying no to?"

Does this yes mean you are saying no to free time, mental space, a chance to catch up on chores, being present for bedtime, or your usual workout? Or, on the other hand, are you saying no to boredom, monotony, or staying in your comfort zone? Every yes comes with a trade-off, whether you consciously choose it or not. The real issue arises when we don't stop to make this calculation. It's perfectly fine to skip a workout or sacrifice some downtime for something meaningful, but if you're constantly saying yes without considering the cost, you may end up feeling stretched thin or even resentful. Before committing, take a moment to assess how this yes fits into your life, how it aligns with your purpose, and whether you're truly okay with what you're giving up in return.

Coaching Notes: Isla's Story

When Isla first came to me for coaching, she felt utterly lost. She had built a career she loved, one she had worked tirelessly to grow in, but life had become overwhelming. She was barely keeping her head above water. The loss of a parent, the breakdown of her relationship, a child with additional needs, and the absence of family support nearby had left her drained. On top of it all, she had always been the person others relied on: the strong one, the helper, never the one to ask for help herself.

She had heard me talk about natural strengths and talents before, but in that moment, her strengths felt like weaknesses. All she saw was someone who was stretched thin, constantly prioritizing others, and feeling increasingly resentful of it. The weight of responsibility was suffocating. She wished she could be like those people who set boundaries with ease, and who asked for help without guilt.

Isla and I worked together to reconnect her with her true strengths and talents. She began to see that her deep sense of responsibility and service – qualities she had always viewed as burdens – were in fact incredible gifts. Coupled with her determination and drive for achievement, these traits had propelled her forward and allowed her to navigate immense challenges. But through our conversations, she realized that her deep need to please others was undermining the very strengths that made her who she was. Instead of being a source of fulfilment, it had become an obligation, leaving her own needs neglected.

Together, we explored practical strategies to help Isla set boundaries, ones that felt natural and aligned with her values, rather than rigid or solely self-focused. She came to understand that people aren't always aware of what we need unless we tell them, so we set a goal: she would ask two people she deeply trusted for help and have an honest conversation with her boss about the personal struggles affecting her work. She also committed to doing something just for herself, despite her long list of responsibilities. Because sometimes, making room for yourself isn't about finding time; it's about deciding that you deserve it. Isla's generous spirit wasn't lost in these adjustments. Instead, she discovered that caring for herself didn't take away from what she gave to others, it made her stronger, more present, and more fulfilled. As she put it:

"I've got a long way to go before I find the balance I need in my life. But I'm learning to think before I commit, I'm practising saying no, I'm valuing my needs, and I'm finally allowing myself to ask for help."

✏Activity: Breaking Free From People Pleasing

Step 1: Recognize your patterns

Take a moment to reflect on your own experiences with people pleasing. Sit with your favourite hot drink and your journal, and try to answer the following questions honestly:

- When was the last time you said yes to something you didn't want to do?
- What was your motivation for saying yes? For example, fear of disappointing someone, avoiding conflict, or seeking approval.
- How did you feel afterwards? Resentful? Overwhelmed? Drained?

Now, think about a time when you said no to something. How did that feel in comparison?

Step 2: Identify your people-pleasing type

Revisit the personality-based people-pleasing tendencies outlined earlier. Which type(s) resonate most with you?

Achiever: overcommitting to prove your worth
Thinker: overexplaining or avoiding confrontation
Connector: prioritizing others' needs at your own expense
Impactor: feeling responsible for others' success
Believer: struggling to say no out of a sense of duty
Explorer: saying yes to everything out of FOMO (fear of missing out)

How does your dominant type influence your choices and behaviour?

Step 3: Set your personal boundaries

Use these prompts to define boundaries that work for you:

- Time limits: how many commitments per week feel manageable for you? How much time can you give to certain types of commitments?
- Emotional energy: what kinds of requests drain you the most? How can you reduce, or at least contain, them? Who do you need to talk to about this?
- Pre-decided limits: what is one rule you can set for yourself to protect your time and energy? For example, "I won't check work emails after 7pm" or "I'll say no to weekend plans if I already have two commitments that week".

Step 4: The "yes/no" trade-off exercise

Before agreeing to something new, ask yourself, "If I say yes to this, what am I saying no to?"

- Write down a recent commitment you made that left you feeling drained. What did saying yes to that take away from your life? For example, sleep, family time, relaxation, or exercise.
- Now, think of a request you might receive in the near future. Before answering, pause and ask yourself the same question. What will your answer be?

Final challenge: for the next week, commit to pausing before saying yes. Try setting at least one small boundary and notice how it makes you feel.

Key Takeaways

Self-sabotage is like being stuck in a desert: draining, frustrating, and keeping you from growth. But recognizing these patterns gives you the tools to escape and build a life aligned with your strengths and purpose.

We commonly self-sabotage in four ways:

- **Impostorism:** that nagging voice saying you're not good enough? It's normal, but not the truth. Impostorism shows up in different forms: perfectionism, overworking, needing all the answers, or struggling to ask for help. The key? Recognizing your unique value, reframing self-doubt, and embracing growth.
- **Fixed mindset:** believing your abilities are set in stone keeps you playing small. A growth mindset, on the other hand, sees challenges as opportunities to develop. Shift your perspective by adding "yet" to your self-talk, focusing on progress over perfection, and embracing mistakes as learning moments.

- **Comparison:** measuring yourself against others robs you of joy and purpose. Social media fuels this trap, making other people's lives seem shinier than they really are. The solution? Stay in your lane. Celebrate others, reject the scarcity mindset, and remind yourself that nobody can do what you do quite the way you do it.
- **People pleasing:** saying yes when you mean no, overcommitting, or seeking validation through being "helpful" comes at a cost. True generosity is a choice, not an obligation. Set boundaries, pause before agreeing, and remember that protecting your energy doesn't make you selfish – it makes you stronger.

The antidote to self-sabotage isn't becoming someone you're not. It's growing into the person you were always meant to be. Recognize these patterns, shift your mindset, and step into your true potential.

Chapter Seven

The Forest

Clarify What Matters Most

Almost every day, I take my dog to the local park, where huge trees have stood for decades, some even for centuries. Their branches stretch wide, their leaves are full, and they seem unshakable, standing tall no matter the season. At first glance, you might assume their strength comes from their height, their size, or even how full their leaves are. But the most vital part of the tree – the part we rarely think about – is the roots.

Beneath the surface, an entire network of roots anchors the tree deep into the earth. These roots draw up the nutrients and water it needs to survive, provide stability during storms, and connect it to the ecosystem around it. If the roots are strong and healthy, the tree will flourish. But if the roots are weak, neglected, or damaged, no matter how full the leaves appear for a time, the tree will eventually wither. The roots either sustain or drain the life above the surface.

Now, think about your own life.

Most people measure success the way we first judge a tree: by what's visible. We look at achievements, career progress, relationships, and social status. We assume that if these external markers are thriving, the person must be thriving too. But, just like a tree, what truly sustains a person is hidden beneath the surface.

That invisible root system? It's your values.

Your values are what anchor you, nourish you, and provide stability in times of uncertainty. They guide your decisions, shape your identity, and determine whether the life you're building is truly fulfilling or just outwardly impressive. When your actions align with your values, you grow strong, resilient, and full of life. When they don't, you may look fine on the outside, but inside, something is off, you feel unsettled, disconnected, or even lost. And just like a tree with weak roots, it might take a storm, a crisis, a major life change, or even just a deep moment of reflection for you to realize that something beneath the surface needs attention.

Your Root System: Values

In this chapter, we're going underground. We're going to examine the root system of your life – your values – and make sure they're strong, deep, and capable of sustaining the purpose you're meant to grow into. We'll explore what values are, how to choose them for ourselves, what it feels like to live in alignment with them (and when we're out of sync), the key to living a more meaningful life, and how to take action to ensure our lives reflect the values we've chosen.

So many books on career and purpose focus on talents and skills, and some may mention values, but I want to take it further. I want to help you build a root system that sustains you in every season. A clear, intentional set of values that not only grounds you but also propels you towards your purpose. A good life becomes a great life when it's anchored in values that truly matter. So, let's bring the hidden work of the roots to the surface, making them stronger, clearer, and more focused than ever.

I haven't found a better definition of values than bestselling author and motivational coach Brené Brown's: "A way of being or believing that we hold most important."[1]

Let's break this down. "A way of being or believing" means that values aren't just things we know or agree with in theory. Values are, in many ways, abstract constructs that we make real by living them out. They serve as a guiding map or code, shaping how we choose to live. "That we hold most important" emphasizes that while there are many things that could be considered valuable, we must decide what truly matters most to us. More on this later.

But why do they matter? Well, values matter for a whole variety of reasons. First, your values act as an internal decision-making compass for your life. When faced with choices, big or small, they provide clarity and consistency. When you have a strong sense of your values, your decisions become more aligned with your true self, rather than being swayed by external pressures or short-term rewards.

Second, your values help you build resilience when life gets tough. When challenges arise, they serve as a source of strength. They provide a sense of stability and direction when the external world feels uncertain or overwhelming. Research shows that living in alignment with our values boosts our mental health, adding a protective measure against anxiety and depression.[2] Your values help you stay grounded, offering clarity on how to navigate difficult situations in a way that aligns with who you are. You place your values like a stake in the ground, giving you security and a clear sense of purpose, no matter how chaotic the world around you may seem.

Your values help you to live an authentic life. When you live in alignment with them, you show up as your true self. They encourage authenticity, ensuring that your actions reflect who you truly are and what you stand for. This leads to greater confidence, self-respect, and a sense of peace because you are not compromising your core beliefs.

Finally, living according to your values brings a sense of purpose and motivation.[3] When your actions are congruent with your beliefs, you experience greater fulfilment and a sense of meaning. This is because rather than merely reacting to life, you are actively creating it based on what truly matters to you.

What Are Your Core Values?

Although the 1980s saw a big push for individuals and workplaces to define their values, the idea itself is far from new. Ancient Greek and Roman philosophers like Aristotle, Seneca, and Marcus Aurelius all had their own lists of virtues to guide their lives. Even Benjamin Franklin, one of the Founding Fathers of the United States, created a system based on 13 core virtues, including industry, justice, and humility, to help him live with intention.[4] Clearly, living according to a set of values has long been recognized as a path to a purposeful life.

The challenge, however – and even Franklin clearly struggled with this as he needed 13 of them – is that we're not always good at defining our personal values. We know the buzzwords, but which ones truly matter to us? With so many competing values, all seemingly important, how do we choose? Well, as hard as it may be, we need to keep the list short. Productivity expert James Clear suggests identifying no more than five core values,[5] while Brené Brown takes it even further, recommending just two.[6] Their reasoning is simple: if *everything* is a priority, *nothing* is a priority.

This echoes the wisdom of philanthropist and entrepreneur Warren Buffett's 5/25 Rule,[7] which offers a practical approach to focusing on what truly matters. In the original story, Buffett's pilot asked him how to focus on the most important things in life. Buffett advised him to list his top 25 goals – a process we could apply to identifying our values. Then, he instructed him to circle the five most important ones, those that truly defined his core focus and direction. All sounds pretty obvious so far. The twist? Buffett told him that the remaining 20 goals should become his "avoid at all costs" list – not because they weren't important, but because they could distract from what mattered most. In this way, the "good" can be the enemy of the great, pulling us away from our core priorities, spreading our energy too thin, and ultimately compromising our commitment to what truly defines us.

This principle applies to values just as much as it does to goals. Let me give you an example. Sam's top five values are family, integrity, learning, adventure, and travel. On his "long list", he also included wealth and loyalty. When offered a job that allows him to work overseas and study at the same time, it seems like the perfect fit for his core values. But then his current employer offers him a significant pay rise to stay, explaining how hard he would be to replace – appealing to his values of wealth and loyalty. Without a clear sense of his top priorities, Sam could easily be swayed by a tempting but ultimately misaligned option. It's not that wealth and loyalty aren't important; they just aren't his *most important* values.

And when *everything* is a priority, *nothing* is a priority.

It's also important to recognize that your values are yours to define. No one else – not your family, your upbringing, or even your life partner – gets to decide them for you. I once worked with Claire, who struggled to include creativity in her top five values. She felt an unspoken external pressure, possibly from childhood influences, to dismiss it as too "frivolous" or not "worthy" enough. But deep down, she knew that creativity was a non-negotiable value in her life, and acknowledging it allowed her to fight for more space for it in her daily life. No one but her could define her values.

Your values are your compass, guiding your decisions, shaping your path, and keeping you aligned with what truly matters. To navigate life with clarity, you need to know what they are. You need to know where your North is.

Activity: Set Your Compass – Identify Your Core Values

In this activity, we'll use a process inspired by Warren Buffett's 5/25 method to help you identify your most important values. Here's how you'll do it:

Step 1: Review the values list

You'll find a list of values included at the end of this activity (or you can find similar lists online). Read through the list carefully.

Step 2: Categorize the values

As you go through the list, sort each value into one of three categories:

- Very important to me
- Somewhat important to me
- Not very important to me

Step 3: Narrow down your top values

Once you've sorted your values, go back to the "very important to me" category. From this set, narrow your list down to just five values (maximum). These will be your core values.

Tip: if you're struggling to choose, you can combine related values under one heading. For example, "Family" and "Friends" could be combined as "Relationships".

Step 4: Add any missing values

If you feel like something is missing from the list, feel free to journal your own values that resonate with you.

Accountability	Excellence	Joy	Safety
Achievement	Fairness	Justice	Security
Adaptability	Faith	Kindness	Self-discipline
Adventure	Family	Knowledge	Self-expression
Altruism	Financial stability	Leadership	Self-respect
Ambition	Forgiveness	Learning	Serenity
Authenticity	Freedom	Legacy	Service
Balance	Friendship	Leisure	Simplicity
Beauty	Fun	Love	Spirituality
Belonging	Future generations	Loyalty	Sportsmanship
Career	Generosity	Making a difference	Stewardship
Caring	Giving back	Nature	Success
Collaboration	Grace	Openness	Teamwork
Commitment	Gratitude	Optimism	Time
Community	Growth	Order	Tradition
Compassion	Harmony	Parenting	Travel
Competence	Health	Patience	Trust
Confidence	Heritage	Peace	Truth
Connection	Home	Perseverance	Understanding
Contentment	Honesty	Personal fulfilment	Uniqueness
Contribution	Hope	Power	Usefulness
Cooperation	Humility	Pride	Vision
Courage	Humour	Recognition	Vulnerability
Creativity	Inclusion	Reliability	Wealth
Curiosity	Independence	Resourcefulness	Wellbeing
Dignity	Integrity	Respect	Wholeheartedness
Diversity	Intuition	Responsibility	Wisdom
Environment	Job security	Risk-taking	
Equality			
Ethics			

The Values Gap

In life, there's a profound sense of dissonance that arises when we fail to live in alignment with our values. This misalignment can lead to a deep inner conflict, one that many people unknowingly endure day in and day out. Anyone else love a good whistleblower or cover-up movie? *Erin Brockovich*, *The Insider*, *The Mauritanian*, and *The Report* are just a few that come to mind. In each film, a significant wrong has been committed and someone fights to expose the truth, blow the whistle, and seek justice. Often, these wrongs can be described as moral injuries.

Moral injury is a term used to describe the psychological and emotional distress that can result from exposure to morally challenging or ambiguous situations. It is a form of trauma that can result from a violation of someone's beliefs or values, or from witnessing or participating in events that conflict with those beliefs or values. It is not a threat to life, but a threat to one's deeply held beliefs and trust.[8] It occurs when we are forced to act against what we believe is right, or when we see ethical lines being crossed over and over again. The concept of moral injury was first used to describe the impact of large-scale events like war or terrorism, but it happens in workplaces every day, with real and lasting consequences. Here's a few examples to bring it closer to home:

- Healthcare workers delivering what feels like inadequate care due to unmanageable workloads
- Teachers pressured to prioritize certain students' results over others to meet targets
- Employees asked to cover for a boss's dishonesty or watch workplace bullying go unchallenged
- Companies repeatedly choosing profit over ethics
- Consistently being asked to stay late at work, and repeatedly missing your children's bedtime because of it

These experiences violate our internal moral boundaries, leading to stress, frustration, and burnout. Many of the people I've worked with don't realize that the root cause of their exhaustion isn't just workplace pressure – it's the feeling of living out of alignment with their values. While this misalignment may not be our fault, recognizing it is our responsibility. The challenge is not just identifying moral injury when it happens, but deciding what we're going to do about it.

I remember exactly where I was when I realized my workplace no longer aligned with my values. It was one of those "aha!" moments: an epiphany that made a tough decision inevitable. Up until that point, I had genuinely enjoyed so much about my work. I had countless opportunities to use my strengths, to develop people and ideas and watch them grow into something great. I worked alongside a group of fun, committed colleagues – people I also considered friends. In fact, I've come to realize that friendship is a core workplace value for me. I don't want to just coexist with colleagues; I want to work with people I trust and care about. And as a leader, I want to invest in people beyond just their job descriptions.

But over time, I began to see that not everyone shared that perspective, and that's okay, there's no judgement here. Still, I couldn't ignore the growing feeling that I was on the outside looking in. While I had a desire to build strong, trusting relationships at work, others did not necessarily have the same priority. And standing in reception that day, I finally owned the truth: something had shifted. My values no longer lined up the way they once had. Some of that was on me and some of it was just circumstance, but ultimately, my internal compass felt off and I knew it was up to me to do something about it. So much had been good, but it was time to take all I had learnt, all I had enjoyed, and make a change.

How Aligned Is Your Life?

You may not be experiencing full-blown moral injury, but you might still feel a disconnect between your values and your daily life. That's why it's so important to pause, reflect, and make the necessary adjustments. Defining your values isn't enough if your actions don't align with them. And the people who take the time to do this make the most progress towards a life of purpose. Take our friend Benjamin Franklin and his 13 values (which we have all agreed is too many). After making his list, he would take a single virtue at a time and reflect on how well his life was representing that desired value in reality. He reflected, recorded his answer, and also shared his progress with others. Now, Franklin by no means achieved perfection in these areas, but there are lessons to be learnt from his process. He clearly knew what his values were, he took the time to see if he was living a life that reflected them, and then did his best to shift his behaviours so that they were increasingly in alignment with his life priorities.

Coaching Notes: Anneliese's Story

When Anneliese came for coaching, she wasn't in crisis, life was "okay". She was happily married with children and enjoyed her job, but she sensed that things could be better. She hoped that by understanding her unique strengths and making some intentional changes, she could create a life that felt more fulfilling. Together, we explored her strengths and weaknesses, but the real turning point came when we focused on defining her values. Anneliese had never been through this process before, and while narrowing it down to just five core values was a challenge, it proved to be transformative.

One of her top values was family. As she reflected on her life through this lens, she realized that her demanding work schedule left her with little time to connect with her children on long days. This misalignment with her values felt deeply unsettling. Bravely, she approached her employer to discuss adjusting her working hours. Expecting a firm no, she was surprised when her request was accommodated.

But Anneliese knew there was more. A deeper sense of unease remained; she had never fully expressed to her husband just how central family was to her. Originally from Germany but living in the UK, she finally admitted to herself, and then to her husband, that she longed to be closer to home. About a year later, I received an incredible update:

"We moved back to Germany two months ago. I've taken a new role here, and my husband has too. It was a huge undertaking, but that first honest conversation about my values was the spark that set everything in motion. Nothing ventured, nothing gained."

The Walk and Talk Axis

How can we assess whether we're truly living out our values with purpose and intention in our daily lives? I've adapted a framework, originally designed to help companies evaluate their commitment to their values and purpose, to help us do the same on a personal level.[9] Before you have a go at applying it to your own life and circumstances, let's examine it. It's a simple two-by-two matrix with "walk" and "talk" as the two axes.

Walk (x-axis): living and knowing your values

This measures how much your actions align with your values. It's about real, tangible efforts to embody what you claim to believe: this includes understanding your values and making choices that reflect that understanding.

- High walk ⟶ You deeply understand and consistently act on your values

- Low walk ⟶ You don't know your values well and/or don't act on them (or you are in environments that cause this disconnect)

Talk (y-axis): expressing your values
This measures how much you communicate or advocate for your values, whether through conversations, social media, activism, or influencing others.

- Low talk ⟶ You don't talk about your values much; you might act on them, but you don't share or advocate for them
- High talk ⟶ You openly share, advocate for, or encourage others to live by certain values

These two axes give us four quadrants and a messy middle:

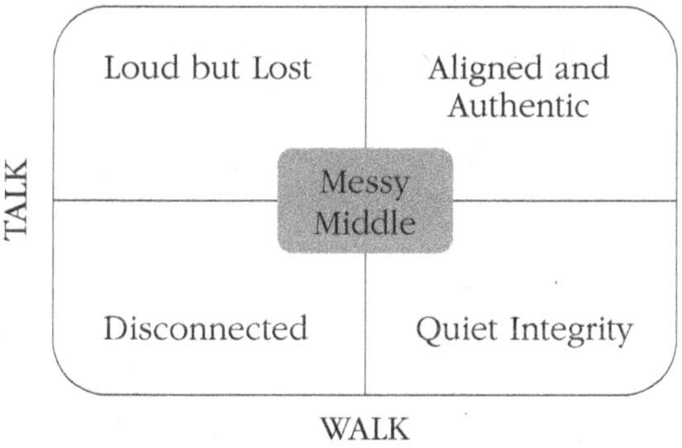

Let's explore the four quadrants.

1. Disconnected (low walk, low talk)
You haven't taken the time to reflect on your values, nor do you express them or live by them. But it's probably not as clear cut as that, and more likely that you go through life making decisions based on what others expect of you or on convenience. You follow trends, societal norms, or the status quo without thinking

about what truly matters to you. You find yourself on a career path because it seemed practical or was expected of you, but you haven't really reflected on what you're passionate about or what aligns with your deeper values.

2. Loud but lost (low walk, high talk)

You talk about your values but don't actively live by them. You advocate for causes or speak passionately about your beliefs, but your actions don't reflect those values. You want to stand by your beliefs, but you struggle with follow-through. It's hard to hear, but maybe it's true: you voice support in meetings for the importance of family, work-life balance, and employee wellbeing, but you don't follow through when it matters. Perhaps you send late-night emails, encourage others to stay late to finish projects, or consistently take on more work without considering the strain it places on your team.

3. Quiet integrity (high walk, low talk)

You live by your values but don't openly talk about them. You lead by example, but you aren't vocal about your beliefs or values. You regularly volunteer your time, help friends or family in need, or donate to causes that are important to you. But you don't seek recognition or share these actions with others. You just do it because it feels right. At work, you prioritize work-life balance by ensuring your team isn't overworked and take time for yourself, but you don't make a public point about it. You just quietly practise balance and integrity, hoping others will take notice by example. You may be hesitant to share out of humility or fear of judgement.

4. Aligned and authentic (high walk, high talk)

You fully understand your values and consistently live by them, while also openly advocating for them and encouraging others to follow suit. You actively live in alignment with your values –

whether that's family, sustainability, honesty, kindness, or fairness – and candidly share and advocate for them. You walk your talk, inspiring others by both living your values and talking about them. For example, perhaps you prioritize work-life balance not just for yourself, but for your team as well. You genuinely believe that taking time to rest and recharge improves productivity and overall wellbeing, so you not only talk to your team about their welfare but also set boundaries to ensure that your work doesn't take over your life.

Messy middle

We've also got the all-important "messy middle" – that space where you might be aware of your values, but there's a gap between what you say and what you do. You might try to live by your values but struggle with inconsistency, or you express your values but don't always back them up with your actions. It's an in-between phase, where you're still figuring out how to integrate your values more fully into your life and work. This section is important because it shows that life isn't always black and white, and it's normal to be in a stage of growth and refinement. However, it's crucial to recognize the messy middle for what it is – not an excuse to avoid facing up to areas where you might not be fully aligned yet, but an honest acknowledgement that you're actively working through it.

Use this next activity as a diagnostic tool to recognize what feels right, what doesn't, and where change is needed. Time for your journal.

Activity: Align Your Compass

You've already identified your five core values, and now it's time to assess how well they show up in your life. This exercise will help you reflect on the alignment between what you believe, how you live, and how you express those values to others.

Step 1: Score your alignment

For each of your five values, rate yourself on a scale from 1–10 for both walk (how well you live by this value) and talk (how openly you express or advocate for this value). Be as honest as you can.

- Walk (living your values): to what extent do your daily actions reflect this value? (1 = rarely, 10 = always)
- Talk (expressing your values): how often do you communicate or advocate for this value? (1 = never, 10 = frequently)

Example:

Value: family
Walk score: 8 (I prioritize family time and set boundaries at work)
Talk score: 4 (I don't often express my belief in work-life balance to others)

Now, repeat this for your five values.

Step 2: Identify your quadrant

Using your scores, plot each value on the walk and talk matrix:

- Low walk/low talk (disconnected): your actions and conversations don't reflect this value much
- Low walk/high talk (loud but lost): you talk about this value, but don't always act on it
- High walk/low talk (quiet integrity): you live this value but rarely express it outwardly
- High walk/high talk (aligned and authentic): you both embody and communicate this value

Which quadrant do most of your values fall into?

Step 3: Reflect

Take a moment to journal on these questions:

- What surprises you? Do any values score lower than expected?
- What gaps do you see? Are there values you deeply care about but struggle to act on?
- How much are outside influences impacting your scores? Is your work or personal life creating an environment that makes it harder for you to live out your values?
- Where do you want to shift? Which values would you like to move into a higher walk or talk category? Pick one at a time.

As we journey on, we will focus on taking action, but even at this stage, ask yourself what's one small action you can take this week to bring one of your values into better alignment?

Remember, the goal isn't perfection, it's progress. This exercise isn't about self-judgement but acknowledging where you stand and how you can move towards a life that truly reflects what matters most to you.

Values: An Expanded Perspective

Values are not just about personal fulfilment. Yes, they allow us to create lives that reflect what matters most to us, but they also have the potential to connect us to something bigger than ourselves. In the previous chapter, I mentioned how generosity can enhance our own lives, not just the lives of those we give to. I want to expand on that idea by showing how embracing a broadened view of our values – living in a way that positively impacts and serves others – benefits everyone involved. We can use our values to take, or we can use our values to give.

In his ground-breaking book, *Give and Take*, Adam Grant categorizes people into three groups: the givers, the matchers, and the takers.[10] Takers seek to maximize what they can gain from others, matchers aim for a fair exchange, but givers are the rare individuals who contribute selflessly, expecting nothing in return. Adam calls this our "reciprocity style", and his findings around how it impacts our success in life are surprising. Where do you reckon givers fall on the success ladder (in terms of pay, influence, impact, promotion, and satisfaction)? Well, they fall to the bottom. But the funny thing is, they also rise right to the top, too. Takers tend to start strong and wane, and matchers end up somewhere in the middle. So, why do some givers rise to the top while others sink to the bottom? Interestingly, it connects to some of the work we've done in the previous chapter. What distinguishes successful givers from those who get overwhelmed, burnt out, and left behind? The answer is simple: successful givers aren't *purely* selfless – they're what Grant calls "otherish".

Be More "Otherish"

Otherish givers are those that look out for others *and* look after themselves. Grant says, "Many people confuse being nice with being helpful. A successful giver says, 'I don't have to say yes all the time; I'll give when I can have the greatest impact, and I won't let it interfere with my productivity.'"

Grant's research shows that successful givers are not only more others-orientated than their peers, but are also more self-interested. They care about the greater good while also valuing their own needs and interests. These so-called "otherish" givers are both altruistic and ambitious – they approach giving *strategically*. While they're just as generous as purely selfless givers, they've learnt how to navigate a world filled with matchers and takers, ensuring others don't take advantage of them. By including themselves on their priority list, "otherish" givers avoid the risk of "generosity burnout". Selfless givers may seem more generous, always putting others' needs first, but Grant's research and supporting studies reveal that, in the long run, they actually give less. This happens because they eventually run out of energy, time, and resources, simply because they don't take enough care of themselves.

So, when it comes to our values, how do we learn to become "otherish" givers? The key is to avoid seeing values as something to solely serve our own needs. This way, we avoid becoming a record-keeping matcher ("I'm only using my values if it works out for me, too"), and instead strategically use our core values as a guide to help us to place our generosity in the right places, at the right time.

But being a giver isn't just about success metrics. Developing a generous worldview through our values enhances our wellbeing too. A meta-analysis of 100 studies found that caring for others is directly linked to higher personal wellbeing.[11] Researchers also discovered that a giver's wellbeing is highest when there is a personal connection to their altruism. Put simply, "I want to give in a way that reflects my personal core values".

Beyond that, altruism isn't just good for others, it's good for us. Studies show that "well-doing" acts as a buffer against stress and negative emotions, even improving longevity. In fact, Gallup found that 9 out of 10 people reported an emotional boost from doing things for others.[12]

Still not convinced? Ask yourself this: do you want a good life, or a great one? This might just be the factor that sets your life apart.[13]

Now that we've broadened our view of our values, let's consider what that might look like in practice.

Activity: Share Your Compass

Now that you've identified your top five values and reflected on how well your life aligns with them, it's time to take it a step further. This activity will help you redefine your values in a way that not only serves you but also benefits those around you.

Step 1: Define your values (personal perspective)
For each of your five values, write a short definition that explains what it means to you personally. Consider why this value matters to you and how it shows up in your life.

Example:

- Family: prioritizing time and being present with loved ones, supporting them emotionally, and creating a sense of belonging
- Health: taking care of body and mind through exercise, nutrition, and rest so I can feel my best
- Adventure: embracing new experiences, exploring the world, and stepping outside my comfort zone
- Fairness: treating others with respect, ensuring equality, and advocating for justice

Step 2: Expand your definition ("otherish" perspective)
Now, rewrite each definition with a broader, outward-looking perspective. Ask yourself, "How can I use this value to positively impact others?" Think beyond how it benefits you and consider how it can be a force for good.

Example:

- Family (expanded view): not only supporting my own loved ones but also fostering a sense of belonging for others who may feel isolated, such as new colleagues, neighbours, or community members
- Health (expanded view): taking care of my own wellbeing while encouraging and supporting others to do the same, whether through sharing knowledge, motivating friends, or advocating for healthier workplaces
- Adventure (expanded view): seeking out new experiences and also inspiring others to step outside their comfort zones,

whether by sharing my experiences, planning group adventures, or encouraging others to take positive risks

- Fairness (expanded view): standing up for equality, advocating for those who may not have a voice, and ensuring that the spaces I am part of are inclusive and just

Brilliant work. Now it's time to bring it all together.

Values for Life

So, we've identified our personal values, evaluated how well we're living them, and even explored how they can benefit others as well as ourselves. But how do we sustain them in our daily lives? It requires action. Like Anneliese, we need to make intentional adjustments that align our lives with our values. As we approach the final chapter, we'll reflect on our broader next steps. But for now, let's focus on the small yet meaningful shifts that allow us to lean into our values, and, ultimately, our purpose.

Focus on one value at a time

Trying to overhaul your entire life at once can feel overwhelming. Therefore, choose one core value to focus on and make small, intentional shifts that bring it to life. For example, if creativity is a core value, you might start by setting aside non-negotiable time each week for a creative pursuit. Once this is embedded, you can move on to another value.

Keep it doable

Big, dramatic changes aren't always necessary, or sustainable. Like Anneliese, larger changes might be on the horizon, but you have to start somewhere, now. Look for simple, practical adjustments that align your life with your values. Small, consistent steps create lasting impact. If health is a value, this might mean adding a short daily walk rather than committing to an intense workout routine that feels unrealistic.

Keep it "otherish"

Find a way to ensure living your values has an expansive view. For example, if achievement is a value, you may set ambitious goals and strive for personal success. But an "otherish" approach would involve not only achieving for yourself but also helping others reach their goals. You might mentor someone who's working towards a similar objective or celebrate the achievements of your peers as much as your own. This way, your drive for achievement doesn't just serve you, it elevates the people around you, too.

Track and reflect

Regularly checking in on how well you're living your values keeps you accountable and allows for course correction. You might journal, set reminders, tell someone, or simply pause at the end of each week to reflect: did my actions align with my values? Where can I improve? Tracking progress helps you stay intentional without becoming rigid.

The most important thing at this point is to actually do *something*. Big journeys start with small steps.

✎Activity: Follow Your Compass

It's time to focus on how you can apply your values and develop a purposeful action plan. Small, intentional steps taken consistently will ensure that your values aren't just words on a page but guiding forces in your everyday life.

Step 1: Choose one value to focus on

Look at your list of core values. Which one feels most relevant or in need of attention right now? Write down the value you're focusing on. Consider the definition you made in the previous reflection.

Step 2: Define a small, meaningful action

Keeping in mind the guidelines, come up with a concrete action that:

- Is small and doable: something realistic that fits into your current life
- Aligns with your value: it should clearly reflect what matters most to you
- Has an "otherish" element: consider how this action might also positively impact others
- Is trackable: you should be able to check in on your progress

Step 3: Write your action plan

Use the following template to make your action clear and specific

- My chosen value: [insert value]
- My action: describe your action in one sentence
- Even better if: take your initial idea and improve it
- How it benefits me: describe how this action aligns with your personal wellbeing
- How it benefits others: describe how this action positively impacts others
- How I will track it: note one way to check in on your progress

Here's an example to get you thinking:

- Value: family
- Action: have a no-phone family dinner every Sunday
- Even better if: once a month, we invite a neighbour, friend, or someone who might be feeling lonely to join us, encouraging a sense of community and belonging
- How it benefits me: strengthens my relationships and helps me feel more connected

- How it benefits others: creates meaningful bonding time, deepens family connections, and offers inclusion to those who may not have a strong support system
- How I will track it: I'll check in after a month to see if this habit feels meaningful and sustainable

Step 4: Take the first step

Now that you have your action, take the first small step today. It could be scheduling time, telling someone about your goal for accountability, or simply setting a reminder.

Step 5: Check in and adjust

At the end of the week, ask yourself: did I follow through? How did it feel? What needs adjusting? Journal your reflections.

By consistently taking small steps, you'll not only live in alignment with your values but also strengthen the deep roots that keep you grounded. Just like a well-rooted tree stands firm through life's storms, your values will anchor you, creating a lasting, positive ripple effect in your life and the lives of others.

Key Takeaways

Your values are the hidden roots of your life, shaping your decisions, guiding your actions, and determining whether you feel truly fulfilled or just outwardly successful. They are your foundations. Like a tree, you might appear strong on the surface, but if your values are neglected, life will eventually feel unsteady.

Most of us rarely stop to define our values, yet they influence everything we do. Without clarity, we risk making choices based on expectations, convenience, or short-term rewards rather than what truly matters. That's why identifying your core values is crucial, for they anchor you and guide you towards living with purpose.

Living in alignment with your values means:

- Using them as a compass for decision-making, ensuring your actions reflect what you believe in
- Recognizing when life pulls you out of alignment and making adjustments before burnout, frustration, or regret set in
- Expanding your perspective and understanding that values aren't just about personal fulfilment
- Using them to help you live with purpose, positively impacting others too
- Taking small, intentional steps to reinforce your values daily, ensuring they aren't just abstract ideals

When you live your values, they shape your character, your legacy, and your ability to create a life that's not just good but deeply meaningful and full of purpose.

Chapter Eight

The Lighthouse

Chart Your Next Steps

"When a man does not know what harbour he is making for, no wind is the right wind."[1] *Seneca*

I'm not exactly a natural sailor. Memories of seasickness, capsized kayaks, and one unfortunate run-in with a yacht's boom have convinced me I'm better off sticking to swimming. But I've always loved lighthouses; the way they rise against the horizon, unwavering through storms, casting their light to guide sailors even in the darkest, most uncertain waters. And as you metaphorically set sail into this next season of your life, you're going to need that lighthouse, too. Because without a clear harbour to aim for, even the strongest wind won't carry you where you want to go.

Many articles, podcasts, and books on purpose do a great job of explaining what it is, how it works, and what to look for, but they often stop there. They shy away from the crucial next step: committing to action. They don't ask you to nail your colours to the mast and decide what comes next. This book is different. It's designed to nudge you forward, whether that means taking a small step, making a mid-course adjustment, or charting an entirely new course.

You've already made incredible progress on this journey. You've reflected on your current life, discovered your true strengths and talents, found clues in your best moments, gained a deeper understanding of your weaknesses, explored how you might be holding yourself back, and created a priority list of values. Now it's time to pull all that together and plan your next steps. Whatever move you decide to make, you'll pinpoint it – and start planning for it. At least a little. In this chapter, as you search for the lighthouse beam, you'll pull together everything you've learnt so far to craft a purpose statement for your life. You'll dream a little, imagining some possible life plans, and then use a mapping tool that you can return to time and again, turning big goals into actionable steps.

Your Personal Purpose Statement

Humans have been asking the question, "What am I here for?" for as long as we've been able to reflect on our existence. There are "big" answers to this question – ones shaped by faith, philosophy, and culture. These broader perspectives help us see how our individual story fits into something larger, whether that's a spiritual belief, a societal contribution, or a philosophical framework for meaning. But purpose isn't just about the big picture; it also has a deeply personal dimension – one shaped by our unique experiences, strengths, and values. That's the aspect I want you to focus on, and a personal purpose statement for your life will guide you along the way.

A personal purpose statement is a clear, concise expression of the core values, beliefs, and motivations that guide your actions and decisions. It helps you stay aligned with what truly matters to you and provides direction in both your personal and professional life. It isn't easy to craft, but it's absolutely worth the effort. It separates you from your manager, your best friend, and the person at work that pushes your buttons. It's not about boxing you in, it's about giving you freedom to pursue the most important things. If well crafted, it enables you to focus on the most important things *to you*: if something is not in line with your purpose statement, you will find the confidence to resolutely decline, knowing it's simply not the right thing for you.

When you're clear on your personal purpose, it becomes easier to filter out distractions, avoid people pleasing, and stop chasing goals that don't align with who you are. When life feels uncertain and you find yourself in a season of difficulty and disappointment, your purpose statement acts like the lighthouse, showing you the direction to head in. When the waves of doubt, setbacks, or change threaten to pull you off course, your purpose statement becomes that steady beam of light, cutting through the fog, reminding you of what truly matters *to you*, and guiding you towards the next right step. Your personal purpose statement serves as your inner motivator, giving you focus so that you can move towards the things that matter most. It's the reminder of why you get up in the morning, what drives you forward, and the impact you're here to make. On both ordinary days and challenging ones, it helps you stay focused, determined, and aligned with the life you want to create.

Recently, I led an away day for female leaders at a large multinational organization. Throughout the day, we explored many of the concepts in this book, building up to a powerful final exercise: crafting and publicly sharing their personal purpose statements. It was the first time I'd approached purpose statements in this way. The women were under time pressure, and were asked to quickly put their thoughts into words then share something deeply personal with the group – knowing it wouldn't be their most polished or perfect version.

But when each woman stood up and spoke her purpose out loud, something remarkable happened. You could feel the shift in the room. Confidence grew with every voice, a sense of solidarity emerged, and their purpose statements, though imperfect, suddenly felt more real, and more alive. They weren't just private thoughts anymore; they were something valuable, something to commit to, and something to be proud of.

Yes, it felt high-risk – but the reward was even higher.

I know this because I've been through it myself. Writing my own personal purpose statement was something I first attempted during the Covid-19 pandemic. I was working from home, trying to write a course in response to the growing number of coaching requests I was receiving on this very topic. I knew I couldn't ask others to do something I wasn't willing to do myself, so I sat down to try and articulate my own purpose.

It wasn't easy. In fact, it was far harder than I expected. But that statement has become something I've returned to time and again – helping me navigate decisions, stay aligned with what matters, and course-correct when needed.

Create a Personal Purpose Statement

So, how do we craft a personal purpose statement – one that isn't just a catchy sentence or two with little depth or individuality? Here's how to create a meaningful and valuable personal purpose statement that brings together all of your hard work throughout this book.

Come back to your true strengths

Your unique talents and strengths are the foundation of your purpose. These aren't just skills or abilities; they are the core elements of who you are. Think of them as your character DNA, shaping the way you contribute to the world. Reflect on moments in your life when you've felt truly engaged, energized, or in flow. These are often the times when you've been operating at your best, and they can provide critical clues about your purpose. You've already done some fantastic work on creating language around your unique strengths.

Identify what drives you

Beyond strengths, consider what fuels your passion. What makes you excited to get out of bed in the morning? What causes or issues do you feel a deep connection to? What are some of the highlights of your day, or the peak moments of your life? Whether it's creating change, serving others, or fostering growth, identifying what lights you up is essential for making your purpose statement authentic and inspiring. Think back over the work you did on your favourite moments so far in life, and the threads that developed from that work. Think too about the roles you play in life, and which matter most to you.

Connect with your values

Your values act as a compass for your purpose. What principles guide your decisions and behaviour? Whether it's integrity, creativity, family, or freedom, your values will help define the lens through which you see the world – and ultimately, the impact you want to have. Make sure your purpose statement aligns with what you truly value, not just what you *think* you should value. You should have a final top five values from the work you've already completed.

Keep it open

Your purpose statement isn't meant to be set in stone. However, if written with flexibility in mind, it already allows for growth and adaptation as seasons and situations change. Life is constantly evolving, and so are you. It's completely normal for your purpose to develop over time. It's not so much that your purpose changes, it's more that the assignment does. Think of your purpose statement as a living document, one that evolves as you grow, learn, and experience new things. The key is to keep it close, revisit it often, and adjust it as needed. What matters most is creating a statement that resonates with you in this season of life, right now.

It should stretch you

Your purpose statement, much like a company's mission statement, shouldn't feel entirely achievable. It should go beyond where you are, representing an ideal of how you would like to live. "Quite a good leader" or "sometimes a generous friend" just don't cut it. It should inspire you to stretch beyond your current limitations, challenging you to grow. It represents an ideal version of yourself, the way you *want* to show up in the world, even if it feels a little out of reach. By pushing you beyond your comfort zone, your purpose statement encourages continuous evolution. It's not about perfection or easy wins, but about setting a bold direction for the person you're becoming, inspiring you to pursue something bigger and more meaningful.

It should pass the "headstone test"

Professor and author Victor Strecher suggests that when trying to sum up our life's purpose, it should pass what he calls the "headstone test".[2] To do this, he recommends drawing a small headstone on your paper (underneath your personal statement), writing your name and date of birth, and then for the date of death, writing "today". The idea is to ask yourself this: what would you want people to say about you at your memorial service? While this exercise might feel a bit extreme, it serves as a powerful reminder. If we aren't living with our ultimate legacy in mind – if our purpose isn't aligned with how we want to be remembered – we risk pursuing goals and ambitions that lead us far off course.

Now get out your journal and take the time to create this most important statement for your life.

Activity: Your Personal Purpose Statement

It's time to take all the reflections, all the hard work, and all you've learnt about yourself, and compile a short personal purpose statement. Look back over some of the activities you've already completed to help you with this. Aim to include, or at least reflect on, some of the following:

- Your strengths
- Your priorities
- Your favourite activities
- Your values

I'm giving you some guidelines, but I don't want to be too prescriptive with this – it needs to work for you. Once you've had a go at writing a draft, check if it passes your "headstone test". You might like a slightly longer version, or you might want to then get it down to a shorter sentence so that you can remember it. Here are a few examples to spark your creative juices (but remember there's no set way to do it).

Example 1 (My current personal purpose statement)
To bring my all to every role I play – as a wife, mother, friend, and more – bringing joy and energy to every room I enter. To love people through communication that inspires and empowers them to discover their purpose. Rooted in my faith, I strive to leave the world a little fairer and more encouraged than I found it, making a lasting impact on my family, community, and beyond.

In short: wholehearted wife, mother, and friend – bringing joy, energy, purpose, faith, and impact.

Example 2
I lead with integrity, fostering honesty and transparency while making mindful, sustainable choices for both my health and the environment. As a deep thinker, I guide my team with clarity and vision, creating an atmosphere of peace where everyone can thrive. My purpose is to inspire positive change in the world and those around me.

In short: integrity-driven leader, fostering honesty, sustainability, clarity, peace, and positive change.

Example 3
To be a dedicated parent, always present and available for my family. I strive to serve those I care about, helping them grow and thrive. I'm committed to nurturing relationships, making time for my loved ones, and using my creativity to bring joy to our lives.

In short: dedicated parent, present, supportive, nurturing relationships, fostering growth, creativity, and joy.

Now that you've worked on your personal purpose statement, it's time to picture what a life aligned with it could look like. When asked to reimagine our lives, we often default to safe, familiar choices. Daily responsibilities can take over, leading us to settle for a version of life that falls short of one that makes us truly happy. But I want you to imagine a life beyond that.

(Re)learning to Dream

These days, I spend most of my time coaching and developing adults, but every now and then I get the opportunity to step back into the classroom and work with younger students. One of my favourite passion projects in recent years was working with a group of sixth form students who were preparing for their next chapter. I was invited to run an intensive version of the principles in this book, tailored for 17- and 18-year-olds. And while I expected their enthusiasm, there was one thing that struck me deeply, and something I rarely see in my work with adults.

They knew how to dream.

When asked to imagine their future, they embraced the possibilities. They eagerly designed different life plans; some practical, others wildly ambitious. They weren't worried about filtering their ideas, questioning whether they were too bold or unrealistic. They weren't concerned with being seen as "too much". Instead, they allowed themselves to explore, expand, and create freely. In a safc and encouraging space, they acknowledged their dreams without fear of judgement or failure.

But what about you?

If you're like many adults, you've probably learnt to filter your dreams, scaling them down until they feel safe, practical, and achievable. I know this has been true for me, too. As a little girl, I had all sorts of ambitions – teacher, yes, but also prime minister (my parents definitely thought I was bossy enough), author, or television presenter. While I may have publicly shared my desire to teach, the other dreams were kept to myself. We worry about being seen as foolish, unrealistic, or naive. We don't want to risk failure, disappointment, or rejection. So we retreat to a place of safety and security instead. For many of us, those dreams don't come true – in fact, only one in four of us end up doing our dream childhood jobs[3] (though this might be for good reason, openings for space cowboys and ballerinas are few and far between). And so, we tinker around the edges of our ambitions, staying within the boundaries of what feels reasonable. Our dreams go back in the box, we close the lid, and continue along the well-trodden path.

But here's the truth: regardless of whether they come true, dreaming is powerful. When we give our imaginations free rein, we can discover alternative future realities. Dreams stretch our thinking, open doors, and remind us that there are always more possibilities than we realize. Imagination allows us to break free from the limits of our present reality. When we envision the future, we can explore different possibilities, anticipate how they might feel, and make more purposeful choices about the path we want to take. Furthermore, allowing ourselves to dream opens the door to creative problem-solving. Rather than settling for the first or most obvious option, dreaming encourages us to push boundaries and imagine better alternatives. But how do we begin, especially as adults who feel out of practice?

Design-Think Your Life

One approach that could help you reimagine your life is design thinking – a method used in problem-solving and innovation that might be just as powerful when applied to our own lives. In the world of work, particularly in product development and innovation, design thinking has transformed the way products and systems are created. Among other things, it encourages experimentation and adaptation rather than assuming a single, fixed solution. Intrigued by its potential beyond engineering and design, product designers Bill Burnett and Dave Evans began to ask, "What if people applied this same process to designing their lives?"[4]

Rather than searching for one "perfect" path, design thinking for life helps us navigate uncertainty with curiosity, creativity, and flexibility. It encourages us to explore multiple possibilities, test ideas through small experiments, and continuously refine our direction – just as a designer would when developing a new product. By shifting from rigid planning to adaptive problem-solving, we can create a future that aligns with our values, aspirations, and evolving circumstances.

To help with this process, Burnett and Evans created the Odyssey Plan,[5] a tool designed to help us imagine multiple possible futures rather than fixating on just one. Instead of mapping out a single life path, you create three distinct versions of your future:

- **Your current life plan:** what does life look like if you continue as you are now?
- **An alternative life plan:** if your current situation were no longer an option, what would you do instead?
- **The "wild card" life plan:** if there were no limitations, judgement, or financial restrictions – if anything were possible – what bold or unconventional path might you explore?

It's essential to approach each of these plans as being equally valid and valuable, rather than ranking them. Each should be a genuine reflection of your interests and aspirations; often, they are far more achievable than you might think.

Once imagined, don't just leave these plans on paper. Fully explore, question, and reflect on them, testing and refining them. This process involves actively engaging with each plan and asking yourself questions about how it aligns with your values, goals, and desires. You might conduct experiments, seek feedback from others, or even take small steps towards exploring these paths in real life. By doing so, you'll refine your thinking and gain a clearer understanding of which direction, or combination of directions, resonates most with you.

But it's important that for now you focus on this key point: this process isn't about simply choosing the "right" one; in fact, it's not about choosing at all. It's about expanding your thinking and giving yourself *permission to dream*. Something powerful happens when you allow yourself to explore different versions of your future. As you consider how each path makes you feel and what elements resonate most, you may uncover unexpected possibilities – ones you wouldn't have seen if you had only focused on a single direction.

So, what would happen if you let yourself dream again? If you allowed yourself to be unfiltered, unapologetic, and unafraid?

Coaching Notes: Imani's Story

Imani came to me through a company initiative that offered employees the opportunity to work with me for personal development. At the time, Imani was working in social media, and life was ticking along just fine. "I wasn't loving work, but I also wasn't hating it," she explains. I pointed out that while feeling okay might seem comfortable, it can also be a dangerous place to stay. It's easy to settle, accept the status quo, and start thinking smaller instead of bigger.

Together, we explored alternative pathways for her future. The first was staying exactly where she was, continuing in social media at her current company. The second was a pivot, moving to a larger company where she could collaborate with other creatives instead of being the lone in-house specialist. The third was bold – leaning fully into her side hustle of making bespoke jewellery. Some of her friends had already bought her designs, and deep down she dreamed of turning it into a business. She imagined using her social media expertise to build a brand with a strong story and a focus on sustainability.

We explored her strengths, values, and the kind of life she truly wanted. She longed to slow down, move away from the hustle, and create ethical, sustainable pieces. The idea both excited and terrified her, as she had no idea where to begin. Then, life threw her a curveball – something she never wanted but ultimately needed: Imani was made redundant.

From that painful moment, her small business was born. "I was devastated to lose my job," she admitted, "but the work I had done on my strengths, values, and dreams gave me the courage to take the leap. I learnt to embrace the uncertainty, and asked myself, 'what's the worst that can happen?'"

Now, a few years down the line, each new season of her work is highly anticipated. She's making a happy living, and she's never looked back.

That's the power of a dream.

✏Activity: Purpose Pathways

Let's take the core principles of design thinking and intentionally apply them to your life in a way that aligns with your purpose. Time for your journal.

Step 1: Imagine your three purpose-driven paths

Take a paper and pen, and – allowing yourself plenty of time to dream – fully explore three versions of your life, each grounded in your strengths, values, and purpose (your purpose statement will help you to do this):

- **The aligned path:** if everything continued as it is, but you fully leaned into your strengths and values, what would your life look like? What small adjustments would make it even more fulfilling?
- **The pivot path:** if life threw a curveball (such as job loss or a major transition), how could you pivot while staying true to your purpose? What strengths would help you navigate change?
- **The bold path:** if fear, failure, and judgement weren't factors, what would you do? What version of your life would push you to your full potential?

Step 2: Consider your strengths and values

Now that you've imagined different possibilities, consider:

- What common themes emerge?
- Which version excites you most?
- What opportunities can you see?
- How do your strengths and values naturally support these visions?
- How would you sum up how this path makes you feel?

Step 3: Overcome inner barriers

What self-limiting beliefs, fears, or external pressures might hold you back from pursuing the path that feels most fulfilling? What problems can you foresee? Which of these fears and beliefs are real, and which are imagined? How can you shift your mindset to move forward with confidence?

Step 4: Explore and experiment

It's not yet time for action – this activity is about allowing yourself to imagine. What adaptations and tweaks can you make to the paths you've planned out to improve them further? Rather than making huge changes all at once, what small, low-risk steps can you take to test your purpose?

Step 5: Reflect

Take some time to sit with your thoughts and emotions. You might even want to write down any reflections or statements that come up during this process. You may experience a range of feelings: unease, excitement, nervousness, and more. As you explore these three pathways, what stands out? How does the bold path differ from the aligned path? What insights has the bold path revealed about your heart's desires? What possibilities or opportunities do you see in the pivot path? Who should you talk to next in order to take the next step?

Take Action

So, after discovering your true strengths, talents, and values, overcoming self-sabotage, crafting a purpose statement, giving yourself space to dream, and exploring possibilities – what comes next? How do you turn these ideas into tangible action? I have to admit, some days I wish a letter would just appear in the post, spelling out exactly what I need to do for the next 12 months.

"Dear Hannah, this is what you should focus on. Say no to these things. Call this person: it will lead to great things. Reply to that email and ask about such and such. Live here, invest in this, spend your time doing that – and you'll get the best possible outcome."

Wouldn't that be amazing?

But, of course, such letters don't exist. Not just because it's a fantastical idea, but also because *maybe there's no such thing as a single best possible outcome.*

What if a perfect path doesn't exist at all? Perhaps a purposeful life isn't about making one "right" choice but about taking action, learning and adjusting as we go. Maybe there isn't *one* best decision, only steps that lead to new insights, new opportunities, and better and better outcomes over time.

What if, instead of chasing certainty, we gave ourselves permission to try, learn, pivot, and try again? What if we stopped waiting for the perfect plan and instead embraced the idea that, in most cases, action is simply better than inaction?

Taking action creates the possibility of positive outcomes

When we step forward and try, we open the door to new opportunities: something good *could* come from it. Of course, not everything will work out, but one thing is certain: if you don't try, nothing happens at all.

It's also helpful to move beyond black-and-white thinking. Most choices aren't simply success or failure; they exist in a space where every step teaches us something. Even when things don't go as planned, we gain insight, adjust, and move closer to the outcomes we're working towards. Progress isn't always immediate, but action keeps us moving in the right direction.

Taking action strengthens both our courage and confidence
Every time we step forward – regardless of the outcome – we prove to ourselves that we can face fear, navigate challenges, and come out stronger. Over time, we build a track record of resilience, something we can rely on when the next challenge comes.

I love this wisdom, often attributed to bestselling author Dale Carnegie: "Inaction breeds doubt and fear. Action breeds confidence and courage. If you want to conquer fear, do not sit home and think about it. Go out and get busy." Because the truth is, most of the good things in life don't happen without courage.

Taking action puts us back in the driver's seat of our own lives
Too often, we drift through life as passengers, letting circumstances or other people dictate our direction. While there's very little we can truly control, one thing we always have power over is our choice: to take action, or to remain passive and wait. That choice shapes everything. I remember working with someone who, very early in our working relationship, told me that they were thinking of moving on. Ten years later, they were still there. Ask yourself: are you making choices in your life, or are you waiting for life to happen to you?

Taking action is the first step towards building momentum
As the old proverb goes, "How do you eat an elephant? One bite at a time." When I started writing this book, the task felt overwhelming – so big that I wasn't sure I'd ever start, let alone finish. So, I broke it down into manageable chunks: first chapters, then sections within chapters. This approach gave me a sense of progress and kept me moving forward. Each sentence I wrote

built momentum for the next, and eventually all those small actions added up. And clearly, the strategy worked, because here you are, holding the finished product. This book wasn't the result of one big action. It was the result of consistent small actions, stacking up over time until the goal was achieved.

Taking action stops perfectionism in its tracks

As I've already said, perfection isn't achievable anyway. That doesn't mean we shouldn't strive for excellence, but as the saying goes, "Perfect is the enemy of good." But what does that actually mean in practice? How does a recovering perfectionist learn to take action instead of holding out for perfection? A good rule of thumb is to move forward when something feels 70 per cent good enough, because waiting for 100 per cent often means waiting forever. I love how the author Oliver Burkeman puts it:

> "The 70% rule: if you're roughly 70% happy with a piece of writing you've produced, you should publish it. If you're 70% satisfied with a product you've created, launch it. If you're 70% sure a decision is the right one, implement it. And if you're 70% confident you've got what it takes to do something that might make a positive difference to the increasingly alarming era we seem to inhabit? Go ahead and do that thing. (Please!)"[6]

Because the truth is, action – even imperfect action (which actually requires more guts) – is always better than being stuck in hesitation.

Taking action minimizes regret

I can't promise that every decision you make will turn out exactly as you hope, or that you'll never second-guess yourself. But I can tell you this: taking action often leads to fewer regrets than standing still. Through his groundbreaking research on the power of regret, author Daniel Pink found that inaction regrets – the things we *didn't* do – are nearly twice as common as regrets tied to actions we *did* take. What's more, these regrets tend to intensify over time. As we age, we don't dwell as much on the risks we took or the mistakes we made; instead, we are haunted by the opportunities we let pass us by, the dreams we didn't chase, and the conversations we never had.[7]

While no choice guarantees a life free of regret, choosing to act – whether that means pursuing a dream, having a difficult conversation, or stepping outside your comfort zone – at least offers the possibility of growth, learning, and change. In contrast, inaction often leaves only unanswered questions and lingering "what ifs".

How to Take Action

So, hopefully I have convinced you *why* you need to take action. But now comes the real challenge: *how*? How do we bridge the gap between where we are now and where we want to be next? For some of you, this journey has already revealed big shifts that feel obvious and necessary. For others, the path forward isn't as clear yet: it will be more of a nudge-by-nudge process, gradually moving you towards the next chapter of your life with more purpose.

But one thing is certain: if nothing changes, then *nothing changes*. And now that you've committed to living with more intention, staying stuck is no longer an option.

Over the years, through my work in coaching and personal development, I've gathered countless tools to help people get unstuck. This next activity is designed to do exactly that, guiding you through small, actionable steps that will help you progress, bit by bit. I've used this tool in my own life – and still do – and I recommend revisiting it every three to four months to stay on track and keep moving forward.

✎Activity: The Four-Point Pursuit

This exercise is designed to help you take achievable action that moves you closer to the life you imagine. Follow this process every three months to build momentum and stay aligned with your purpose. Get out your journal, and let's begin.

Step 1: Go South ⟶ Reflect on where you've been

Before looking ahead, pause and reflect on the last three months. If you need prompts, check your diary, scroll through your photo roll, or revisit past notes.

Remind yourself of your strengths: who are you at your best? Write down your top three strength types (Achiever, Thinker, Connector, Impactor, Believer, Explorer).

List your achievements: write down everything you've accomplished in this time – big or small, personal or professional. Keep going beyond your first thoughts. Examples include:

- Delivered a great presentation at work
- Decorated the bathroom
- Got a promotion
- Started Couch to 5K
- Finally tackled that tricky email
- Helped my child with exam revision
- Finished reading two books
- Reconnected with old friends

Make this even more meaningful by linking your achievements to your strengths. What qualities helped you succeed?

Step 2: Head North → imagine the future
Now you're going to practise your dreaming. Imagine it's 12 months from today; what does life look like? Write a diary entry in the present tense, as if you're already living that future. Be optimistic, and be bold. No filtering – and no overthinking.

Example:

"The house is on the market, and we've decided on our next location. I've taken on new responsibilities at work, including managing a team. My son has finished his exams and is proud of his effort. I've joined a weekly running group and completed a half marathon. I've read 12 books and seen my friends for drinks every fortnight. My dad has moved into his new retirement flat. We've halved our credit card debt."

This is not a contract, just an exercise in possibility thinking. Let yourself imagine the best version of your life.

Step 3: Go East → Plan your next steps
Dreaming is great, but how do you actually get there? The next 12 months won't look different unless you take specific, measurable steps *in the next three months*. Nothing happens, if nothing *different* happens. Make your action list concrete and realistic, but stretching.

Examples (based on the previous example):

- Redecorate the kitchen and list remaining jobs to prepare the house for sale
- Decide as a family on the top three criteria for choosing a new home

- Talk to my line manager about leadership training
- Take my son out for dinner to check in on his exam stress
- Start a 10K running plan
- Read three books
- Take my dad to see the new retirement flats
- Set a family budget to increase monthly savings

Each step moves you closer to the future you envisioned.

Step 4: Go West ⟶ Expand your horizon

Before you finish, take a step back and revisit steps 2 and 3. Are you playing it too safe? Ask yourself:

- Am I thinking big enough, or am I staying in my comfort zone?
- Am I truly aligning with my values and making a meaningful contribution to the world around me?
- What would 10 per cent braver look like?

Example tweaks:

- Instead of halving credit card debt, clear it completely
- Instead of just reading books, start a book club and help others grow
- Instead of just running 10K, do it for charity
- Instead of waiting for a promotion, mentor someone at work now

Small shifts can make a big difference. Don't just pursue a *good* life – pursue a *great* one.

Short on time? Try the five-minute version

If you don't have time for the full activity, remember that doing something is always better than doing nothing. If you've got just five minutes, try this quick reflection:

- **South:** what's one thing I'm proud of from the last three months?
  Example: started running once a week, even when I didn't feel like it.
- **North:** what's one difference I'd love to see in my life a year from now?
  Example: be able to run a 10K comfortably and feel stronger overall.
- **East:** what's one step I can take in the next three months to move towards that goal?
  Example: follow a structured 5K training plan and schedule three runs per week.
- **West:** what's one small thing I can do for someone else?
  Example: invite a friend to join me for a weekly run to keep each other motivated.

Even small actions create momentum. Take five minutes and set your next step in motion.

Take the Leap

This process isn't a one-time thing, and it's not easy, but it works. It's a proven tool I use in my own life and with the people I coach. Every time I revisit it, I see momentum, progress, and breakthroughs. Commit to doing this every three months to stay focused, adapt, and keep moving towards the life you truly want. When you revisit, take a look at the previous version so that you can see how far you've come and what you might need to adjust for the next period. You don't need to have it all figured out – you just need to take the next step.

Now that you've reflected, dreamed, and planned your next steps, it's time to take the leap towards action. You've got the tools, the roadmap, and the insight to guide you forward. It's not about executing a flawless plan from start to finish; it's about starting and letting momentum build from there. Each small step you take compounds, unlocking new opportunities and giving you the courage to tackle the next challenge.

The truth is, the life you've imagined might be closer than you think. Whether it's a promotion at work, a personal project you've been dreaming of, or simply creating more space for the things that matter most, *action* is the bridge between where you are now and where you want to be. Each time you follow through on one of those small steps – whether it's signing up for that course, sending that email, or simply setting aside time to plan – you're creating the future you've been envisioning.

And here's the key: taking action builds momentum. Once you get going, it becomes easier to *keep* going. It's like getting on a bike – you might feel a little wobbly at first, but with each pedal stroke you move closer to your destination. You'll face bumps in the road, and there may be moments of doubt or fear, but keep going. The more you do, the more confident you'll become, and even when things don't go perfectly, you'll be moving forward.

Now is the time to begin bringing your vision to life. Trust in the process, trust in your ability to adapt and adjust, and – most importantly – trust that with every small step, you're making progress towards the more purposeful life you're looking for.

Key Takeaways

Without action, purpose remains an idea rather than a reality. This chapter has been about moving from reflection to action – bringing together everything you've discovered so far and turning it into practical next steps.

Your personal purpose statement is your lighthouse. It provides clarity when life feels uncertain, helping you filter out distractions, overcome self-doubt, and make decisions that align with what truly matters. When fear or hesitation creeps in, this statement anchors you, reminding you why you started.

To make real progress, you need three things:

- A clear vision of where you're headed
- The willingness to dream
- The courage to take action

To help with this, the Purpose Pathways exercise challenges you to explore three possible versions of your future:

- **The aligned path:** building on your strengths and values to enhance your current trajectory
- **The pivot path**: adapting to unexpected changes while staying true to your purpose
- **The bold path**: imagining what's possible if fear and external expectations weren't holding you back

Once you've mapped out your possibilities, take action by using the Four-Point Pursuit every three months:

- **Go South** ⟶ Reflect on the past three months: your achievements, strengths, and progress
- **Head North** ⟶ Imagine where you want to be a year from now: dream big and be specific
- **Go East** ⟶ Identify tangible, measurable steps for the next three months to move closer to your vision
- **Go West** ⟶ Expand your horizon – are you thinking big enough? Are you playing it too safe? What difference can you make?

Final thoughts

- **Progress comes through action, not perfection:** Taking action – even imperfect action – creates momentum. Waiting for the "perfect" plan often leads to inaction. As Oliver Burkeman puts it, if something is 70 per cent good enough, it's ready to go.
- **Your purpose will evolve – and that's okay:** You don't need to have everything figured out. Purpose isn't about following a rigid, step-by-step plan, it's about taking action, learning from it, and adjusting your course as you go. Progress is built through trial, error, and reflection, not by waiting until you feel fully ready.
- **A year from now, what will you look back on?** Most regrets come from inaction, not action. Research shows we regret the opportunities we didn't take far more than the mistakes we made. A year from now, you'll look back at today and either feel proud that you took action, or regret that you stayed where you were. Which one will it be?

You don't need to have it all figured out – you just need to take the next step.

Afterword

And so, here we are – at the end of the book, but really, still at the beginning of your next chapter.

When writing a book like this, the temptation is to end with an empowering speech – one that declares you now have all the answers, that you're fully equipped to step boldly into a glorious and unique purpose. But life doesn't work like that. You know that, and I know that. Life is unpredictable. It comes with obligations, responsibilities, and unexpected twists and turns. Most of us can't just throw caution to the wind and join the metaphorical circus.

But here's what I *do* hope for you.

I hope you realize that you are made with unique strengths, talents, and ways of seeing the world that no one else can. That within you are ideas, creativity, and perspectives that really matter. Maybe the whole world won't remember your name, but that was never the point. Each of us has the chance to leave a legacy that counts.

I hope you see more of the brilliance within you, and recognize the ways you might be holding yourself back from letting it shine. That you'll notice the wonder in others without it making you feel small or like an impostor. That you'll build boundaries and balance, creating space for your gifts to thrive in a way that's not just good for the world, but also good for you.

And above all, I hope you'll see that it's never too late, that purpose isn't reserved only for the young or the extraordinary but is also found in the ordinary, everyday lives of people like you and me: in the choices we make, in the way we show up, and in the difference we make in the lives of those around us.

Purpose isn't something you *wait for*. It's something you *live*. And now, it's over to you.

Hannah x

Acknowledgements

So many people have encouraged me throughout the process of writing this book. I couldn't have done it alone, and at the risk of leaving someone out, I want to take a moment to thank those who supported me along the way.

First, my deepest gratitude goes to Jesus. Above all else, He gives my life purpose, meaning, and fulfilment. *Soli Deo Gloria.*

My Sam. You are my rock. Your unswerving belief in me, sense of adventure, and secure presence in my life in every season have given me the confidence to pursue a life of purpose. Thank you for your unlimited patience and willingness to listen, and for the countless cups of tea. I love you, always.

Noah, Jude, and Levi – being your mom is my greatest joy. Watching your lives unfold is a gift: Noah, for your inner strength and gentle steadiness; Jude, for your big presence and even bigger heart; Levi, for your thoughtfulness and determination. Amelie, I'm so glad you've joined our family, you are the definition of love, joy, and fun!

Mom, you always believed I'd write a book. Thank you for your deep love and belief in me; you've always said I could do it. This is for you.

Dad, thanks for giving me shoulders. Thank you too for teaching me about hard work and dedication, I hope this book is one way I can honour that example.

Keely, my day one. The best big sister any little sister could ever hope for, you've always wanted more for me than for yourself. I love you.

Alex, thank you for the encouragement and challenge to always dream bigger.

To the rest of the Jennings tribe, I love you all so much, each and every one of you.

To my Miller family, thank you for loving me and letting me join your unit.

To the friends that became family: Jess, Ben, and Solly; James and Becca; Callum and Alice. I love you!

Laura – more than an EA: proofreader, memory jogger, list-maker, daily encourager… truly brilliant. I couldn't have done this without you. Love to David, Han, Debi, and Steve.

James – it all started with a voice note from France. Thank you for saying yes, for sticking with it through the tears and challenges. I love you and I'll always be forever grateful.

Zo, your quiet wisdom and steady support built my confidence more than you know.

To ALL my wonderful friends – from every season of my life – you know who you are, but special mention to Emma, Jo, Mel, Vicky, and Kate in this season. I'm so grateful for all the love, chats, encouragement, and prayers. I have the best friends ever.

Zoë – a special thank you to my dear friend for believing I could do this, encouraging me to take my dream and make it happen. And to all the others who kept asking, "When's the book coming?" – thank you for seeing it before I did.

Thank you to all the mentors and friends that saw potential in me and freely gave wisdom, advice, and encouragement in the early days of my business: especially Nick Harding, Nish Manek, James and Fiona Hill, Tim and Rach Hughes, Marg Bristow, Mary Grinham, Rach Wilson, Kevin Kerley, and Ben Wales.

To my strengths coach besties, Justin and Liz: I am so glad I met you! You have been a constant source of wisdom and friendship since starting out on my own – thank you so much for modelling a purpose-driven way to do work.

Elizabeth, Jasmin, and Fritha – DK dream team! Thank you for your brilliance, edits, and for making this book ten times better.

To the wonderful women in the first Purpose Pursuit focus group – your early feedback shaped this work.

Thank you to the first cohort and all Purpose Pursuit alumni. I get to work with such wonderful, unassuming human beings who have so much to give the world – I hope you know how uniquely brilliant you all are!

And to *you*, the reader – thank you for picking up this book. I hope these pages remind you of what makes you *you*: uniquely and wonderfully made. May they nudge you towards bold dreams, unknown paths, and a life of purpose.

References

Introduction

1. Jill Tomlinson, *The Owl Who Was Afraid Of The Dark* (London: Meuthen, 1968)
2. Victor J Strecher, *Life On Purpose, How Living For What Matters Most Changes Everything* (New York. HarperOne, 2016)
3. Marcus Buckingham, *Love + Work* (Boston, MA: Harvard Business Review Press, 2022)
4. William Damon and Heather Malin, 'The Development of Purpose: An International Perspective', *The Oxford Handbook of Moral Development: An Interdisciplinary Perspective,* Feb 2020, available at: https://coa.stanford.edu/sites/default/files/devel_purpose_intl_persp.pdf (accessed February 2025)
5. J David Creswell, William T Welch, Shelley E Taylor, et al., 'Affirmation of personal values buffers neuroendocrine and psychological stress response', *Psychological Science*, 16(11), 846–851, November 2025, available at: https://journals.sagepub.com/doi/10.1111/j.1467-9280.2005.01624.x (accessed February 2025)

1: The Route

1. Adam L Alter and Hal E Hershfield, 'People search for meaning when they approach a new decade in chronological age', *PNAS*, 17 November 2014, available at: https://doi.org/10.1073/pnas.1415086111 (accessed January 2025)
2. Lindsey Bever, 'Why the most meaningful birthdays end with 9, as in 29 and 39', *Washington Post*, 21 November 2014, available at: https://www.washingtonpost.com/news/morning-mix/wp/2014/11/21/why-the-most-meaningful-ages-end-with-9-as-in-39/ (accessed March 2025)
3. Annie Dillard, *The Writing Life* (London: Picador, 1990)
4. Naina Dhingra, Andrew Samo, Bill Schaninger, et al., 'Help your employees find purpose or watch them leave', McKinsey, 5 April 2021, available at: https://www.mckinsey.com/capabilities/people-and-organizational-performance/our-insights/

help-your-employees-find-purpose-or-watch-them-leave (accessed January 2025)

5. Suwen Lin, Louis Faust, Pablo Robles-Granda, Tomasz Kajdanowicz, Nitesh V Chawla, 'Social network structure is predictive of health and wellness'. *PLOS ONE*, 2019; [14(6)]: e0217264 DOI: 10.1371/journal.pone.0217264
6. Bruce Y Lee, 'Study Finds Less Loneliness Among Those With A Sense Of Purpose', Forbes, 21 January 2024, available at: https://www.forbes.com/sites/brucelee/2024/01/21less-loneliness-seen-among-those-with-a-sense-of-purpose/ (accessed January 2025)

2: The Guide

1. The concept of self-understanding and unique talents features in early writings. As well as Socrates, Aristotle, and Descartes, early biblical writers lean into the concept of individual gifts and talents, such as in Exodus 31:2–5/ Shemot 31:2–5 (Old Testament and To'rah), Peter in 1 Peter 4:10 (New Testament)
2. Sigmund Freud (1856–1939) was the founder of psychoanalysis, a theory of how the mind works and a method of helping people in mental distress. 'Who was Sigmund Freud?' Freud Museum London, n.d., available at: https://www.freud.org.uk/education/resources/who-was-sigmund-freud (accessed November 2024). Jung's work on the shadowside further emphasized the blind spots of our personality. 'Shadow', n.d., available at: https://en.wikipedia.org/wiki/Shadow_(psychology) (accessed November 2024)
3. Peter Flade, Jim Asplund, Gwen Elliot, 'Employees who use their strengths outperform those who don't', Gallup, 8 October 2015, available at: https://www.gallup.com/workplace/236561/employees-strengths-outperform-don.aspx (accessed November 2024)
4. 'Signature Strengths', Via Institute on Character, n.d., available at: https://www.viacharacter.org/research/findings/signature-strengths (accessed November 2024)
5. Martin EP Seligman and Tracy A Steen, 'Positive psychology progress: empirical validation of interventions', *Positive Psychology*, 22 April 2005, pp. 6–9, available at: https://greatergood.berkeley.edu/images/uploads/Seligman-PosPsychProgress.pdf (accessed November 2024)
6. Amy M Anderson, Justina Or, and Kelly R Maguire, 'The relationships between strengths-based teaching practices and students' general, strengths, and academic self-efficacy', *Discover Psychology*, May 2024,

pp. 1, 5, available at: https://link.springer.com/article/10.1007/s44202-024-00171-0 (accessed November 2024)

7. Alex P Linley, Karina M Nielsen, Alex M Wood, et al., 'Using signature strengths in pursuit of goals: Effects on goal progress, need satisfaction, and well-being, and implications for coaching psychologists', *International Coaching Psychology Review*, March 2010, pp. 6–15, available at: https://explore.bps.org.uk/content/bpsicpr/5/1/6 (accessed November 2024)
8. Jim Asplund, James K Harter, Sangeeta Agrawal, et al., 'The Relationship Between Strengths-Based Employee Development and Organizational Outcomes, CliftonStrengths Meta-Analysis', Gallup, May 2015, available to download report at: https://www.gallup.com/cliftonstrengths/en/269615/strengths-meta-analysis-2015.aspx (accessed November 2024)
9. WOBI Inspiring Ideas, 'Marcus Buckingham: Identify Your Strengths', YouTube, 5 December 2013, available at: https://www.youtube.com/watch?v=czsEJGJnPAY&t=33s (accessed May 2025)
10. Tina JC Polderman, Beben Benyamin, Christiaan A de Leeuw, et al., 'Meta-analysis of the heritability of human traits based on fifty years of twin studies', *Nature Genetics*, Vo.47, No.7, July 2015, pp. 702–709, available at: https://www.nature.com/articles/ng.3285.epdf (accessed November 2025)
11. Sarah E Hampson, Lewis R Goldberg, Thomas M Vogt, et al., 'Forty years on: teachers' assessments of children's personality traits predict self-reported health behaviors and outcomes at midlife', *Health Psychology*, January 2006, pp. 57–64, available at: https://pmc.ncbi.nlm.nih.gov/articles/PMC1363685/pdf/nihms2182.pdf (accessed November 2025)

3: The Waterfall

1. The word *poí¯ema* features twice in the New Testament – Romans 1:20 and Ephesians 2:10. Plato, Herodotus, and others discussed the connected word *poiesis* in their writings. The use of the word, and connected words, in the classics is discussed at length in Nathan A Greenberg's paper, 'The Use of poí¯ema and Poiesis', *Harvard Studies in Classical Philology*, 1961, Vol. 65 (1961), pp. 263–289
2. B Niles, 'Note By Note – The Making of Steinway L1037', PBS, 2007, available at: https://www.steinway.com/misc/note-by-note (accessed May 2025)

3. Clare Nickerson, 'Looking-Glass Self: Theory, Definition & Example', *Simple Psychology*, 22 September 2023, available at: https://www.simplypsychology.org/charles-cooleys-looking-glass-self.html#Goffmans-The-Presentation-of-Self-in-Everyday-Life (accessed November 2024)
4. Alex Hutchinson, 'Human Resources', The Walrus, 1 October 2018, available at: https://thewalrus.ca/human-resources/(accessed November 2024)
5. Hannah Miller, The Purpose Pursuit, 'My Story', Episode 32, 28 August 2024, available at: https://open.spotify.com/episode/5fmrtpZWjl0bu2u5cqP0ve?si=fD-Dv7yXT7ONh-OcSYsDlg (accessed December 2024)
6. Volvo, 'Meet The New Volvo EX90', YouTube, 4 September 2024, available at: https://youtu.be/cQX-QXxwGvA?si=PvTlznuv1KhCHjM3 (accessed December 2024)
7. TEDxTalks, 'David JP Phillips: The magical science of storytelling', TEDx Stockholm, TEDx, YouTube, 16 March 2017, available at: https://www.youtube.com/watch?v=Nj-hdQMa3uA (accessed December 2024)
8. Joseph Campbell, *The Hero with a Thousand Faces* (California: New World Library, 2012)

4: The Mountain

1. Elena Mylona and Jonathan Gershuny, 'Time Use Data: What Can Instantaneous Enjoyment Tell Us About Life Satisfaction?, *What Works Centre for Wellbeing: Time Use and Wellbeing*, July 2023, available at: https://whatworkswellbeing.org/projects/time-use-and-wellbeing/ (accessed December 2024)
2. Tait D Shanafelt MD, Colin P West MD PhD, Jeff A Sloan, et al., 'Career Fit and Burnout Among Academic Faculty', *Archives of Intern Medicine,* May 2009, No. 10: [pp. 990–992], available at: https://jamanetwork.com/journals/jamainternalmedicine/fullarticle/415000 (accessed May 2025)
3. Gretchen M Spreitzer and Christine Porath, 'Creating Sustainable Performance', *Harvard Business Review,* Jan–Feb 2012, available at: https://hbr.org/2012/01/creating-sustainable-performance (accessed December 2024)
4. Jim Harter and Amy Adkins, 'Employers Want a Lot More From Their Managers', Gallup, 8 April 2015, available at: https://www.gallup.com/workplace/236570/employees-lot-managers.aspx (accessed December

2024)

5. Beth Axelrod, Helen Handfield-Jones, and Ed Michaels, 'A New Game Plan for C Players', *Harvard Business Review,* January 2002, available at: https://hbr.org/2002/01/a-new-game-plan-for-c-players (accessed December 2024)

5: The Valley

1. Roy F Baumeister, Ellen Bratslavsky, Catrin Finkenauer, et al., 'Bad Is Stronger Than Good', *Review of General Psychology,* 2001, Vol. 5, No. 4, available at: https://homepages.se.edu/cvonbergen/files/2013/01/Bad-Is-Stronger-than-Good.pdf (accessed February 2025)
2. 'Weakness', Oxford English Dictionary, n.d., available at: https://www.oed.com/dictionary/weakness_n?tab=factsheet#15142576 (accessed February 2025)
3. Ben Wigert, 'Employee Burnout: The Biggest Myth', Gallup blog, 13 March 2020, available at: https://www.gallup.com/workplace/288539/employee-burnout-biggest-myth.aspx (accessed February 2025)
4. Tim Tonkin, 'Burnout Hits Record High', BMA blog, 19 July 2022, available at: https://www.bma.org.uk/news-and-opinion/burnout-hits-record-high (accessed February 2025)
5. Herbert J Freudenberger, 'Staff Burn-Out', *Journal of Social Issues,* Winter 1974, Vol. 30, Issue 1, pp. 159–165, available at: https://doi.org/10.1111/j.1540-4560.1974.tb00706.x (accessed February 2025)
6. Saul McLeod, 'Thin-Slicing Judgments In Psychology', Simple Psychology blog, 29 January 2024, available at: https://www.simplypsychology.org/thin-slicing-psychology.html (accessed February 2025)

6: The Desert

1. Pauline Rose Clance and Suzanne Ament Imes, 'The imposter phenomenon in high achieving women: Dynamics and therapeutic intervention', *Psychotherapy: Theory, Research and Practice*, 1978, 15(3), 241–247, available at: www.paulineroseclance.com/pdf/ip_high_achieving_women.pdf (accessed January 2025)
2. Sheryl Sandberg, *Lean In* (New York, Alfred A. Knopf, 2013)
3. Seth Godin, 'Impostor Syndrome', Seth's Blog, 29 October 2017, available at: https://seths.blog/2017/10/imposter-syndrome/ (accessed January 2025)

4. Valerie Young, *The Secret Thoughts of Successful Women: Why Capable People Suffer from the Impostor Syndrome and How to Thrive in Spite of It* (New York: Crown Business, 2011)
5. Dr Carol S Dweck, *Mindset: How you can fulfil your potential* (London: Robinson, 2012)
6. Carol Dweck, 'What Having a "Growth Mindset" Actually Means', *Harvard Business Review*, 13 January 2016, available at: https://hbr.org/2016/01/what-having-a-growth-mindset-actually-means (accessed January 2025)
7. Michael Jordan 'Failure' Nike commercial, available at: https://youtu.be/45mMioJ5szc?si=ydPQYbXWOiDxNV8- (accessed January 2025)
8. 'Hawksmoor Manchester: Diners given £4,500 red wine by mistake' BBC News, 16 May 2019, available at: https://www.bbc.co.uk/news/uk-england-manchester-48292972 (accessed January 2025)
9. Leon Festinger, 'A Theory of Social Comparison Processes', *Human Relations*, 1954, available at: https://journals.sagepub.com/doi/10.1177/001872675400700202 (accessed January 2025)
10. Mai-Lyn Steers, Robert E Wickham, Linda K Acitelli, 'Seeing Everyone Else's Highlight Reels: How Facebook Usage is Linked to Depressive Symptoms', *Journal of Social and Clinical Psychology*, Vol. 33, No. 8, 2014, pp. 701–731, available at: https://www.researchgate.net/publication/267029087_Seeing_Everyone_Else's_Highlight_Reels_How_Facebook_Usage_Is_Linked_to_Depressive_Symptoms (accessed January 2025)
11. Alison Beard and Hailey Magee, HBR IdeaCast, Episode 979, 16 July 2024, available at: https://hbr.org/podcast/2024/07is-people-pleasing-holding-you-back (accessed February 2025)
12. Alison Beard and Hailey Magee, HBR IdeaCast, Episode 979, 16 July 2024, available at: https://hbr.org/podcast/2024/07 is-people-pleasing-holding-you-back (accessed February 2025)
13. Summer Allen, 'The Science of Generosity', Greater Good Science Center at Berkeley, May 2018, available at: https://ggsc.berkeley.edu/images/uploads/GGSC-JTF_White_Paper-Generosity-FINAL.pdf (accessed February 2025)

7: The Forest

1. Brené Brown, *Dare To Lead* (New York: Random House, 2018)
2. Hamdullah Tunç, Paul Graham Morris, Joanne M Williams, et al., 'The

role of valued priorities and valued living on depression and anxiety among young people: A cross-sectional study', *Personality and Individual Differences*, July 2024, Vol. 225, pp. 241–247, available at: https://doi.org/10.1016/j.paid.2024.112680 (accessed February 2025)

3. Shalom H Schwartz and Florencia M Sortheix, 'Values and Subjective Well-Being', in *Handbook of well-being*, E Diener, S Oishi, and L Tay (eds) (Salt Lake City, UT: DEF Publishers, 2018), available at: https://helda.helsinki.fi/server/api/corebitstreams/9a4c0831-ed19-4e7d-889c-1bff700ba1f5/content (accessed February 2025)
4. David G Allan, 'Ben Franklin's "13 Virtues" Path to Personal Perfection', CNN, 1 March 2018, available at: https://edition.cnn.com/2018/03/01/health/13-virtues-wisdom-project (accessed March 2025)
5. James Clear, 'Core Values List', James Clear, n.d., available at: https://jamesclear.com/core-values (accessed March 2025)
6. Brené Brown, 'Living Into Our Values', Brené Brown, n.d., available at: https://brenebrown.com/resources/living-into-our-values/ (accessed March 2025)
7. James Clear, 'Warren Buffett's "2 List" Strategy: How to Maximize Your Focus and Master Your Priorities', James Clear, n.d., available at: https://jamesclear.com/buffett-focus (accessed March 2025)
8. Victoria Williamson, Dominic Murphy, Andrea Phelps, et al., 'Moral injury: the effect on mental health and implications for treatment', *The Lancet*, June 2021, Vol. 8, Issue 6, pp. 453–455, available at: https://www.thelancet.com/journals/lanpsy/article/PIIS2215-0366(21)00113-9/fulltext (accessed February 2025)
9. Christopher P Blocker, Joseph P Cannon, and Jonathan Z Zhang, 'Are Your Company's Purpose Initiatives Working?' *Harvard Business Review*, 6 February 2025, available at: https://hbr.org/2025/02/are-your-companys-purpose-initiatives-working (accessed February 2025)
10. Adam Grant, *Give and Take, A Revolutionary Approach to Success* (New York: Viking, 2013)
11. Jim Clifton and Jim Harter, *Wellbeing At Work*, (New York: Gallup Press, 2021), p. 72
12. Jim Clifton and Jim Harter, *Wellbeing at Work: How to Build Resilient and Thriving Teams* (New York: Gallup Press, 2021)
13. Tom Rath and Jim Harter, *Wellbeing: The Five Essential Elements* (New York: Gallup Press, 2010)

8: The Lighthouse

1. Lucius Annaeus Seneca, 'Letter 71 – On The Supreme Good', *Letters from a Stoic*, 25 December 2018, available at: https://www.lettersfromastoic.net/letter-71-on-the-supreme-good/
2. Victor J Strecher, *Life On Purpose, How Living For What Matters Most Changes Everything* (New York: HarperOne, 2016)
3. 'Childhood Dreams', Legal and General, n.d., available at: https://www.legalandgeneral.com/insurance/life-insurancechildhood-dreams/ (accessed April 2025)
4. Bill Burnett and Dave Evans, *Designing Your Life* (New York: Alfred A. Knopf, 2016)
5. Bill Burnett and Dave Evans, *Designing Your Life* (New York: Alfred A. Knopf, 2016), pp. 80-92
6. Oliver Burkeman, 'Seventy per cent', The Imperfectionist blog, n.d., available at: https://ckarchive.com/bwvu2hghk5m82zf9r552rqtn34kzxxc8 (accessed February 2025)
7. Daniel H Pink, *The Power of Regret: How Looking Backward Moves Us Forward* (New York: Riverhead Books, 2022)